TREATING THE POOR

A Personal Sojourn Through the
Rise and Fall of Community Mental Health

MATTHEW P. DUMONT, M.D

AUTHOR OF *THE ABSURD HEALER*

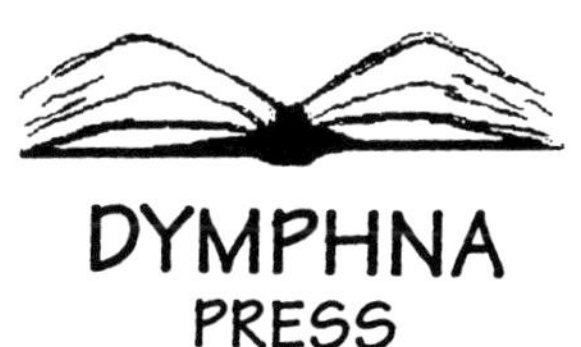

DYMPHNA
PRESS

31 Willow Street
Belmont, MA 02478

Second edition January, 1994

Published by Dymphna Press
Box 44, Belmont, MA 02178

Printed in the United States.

ISBN 0-9634-975-0-2

Library of Congress # 92-97289

Book and cover design: Jane Cook
Front and back cover illustrations: Norma Dumont

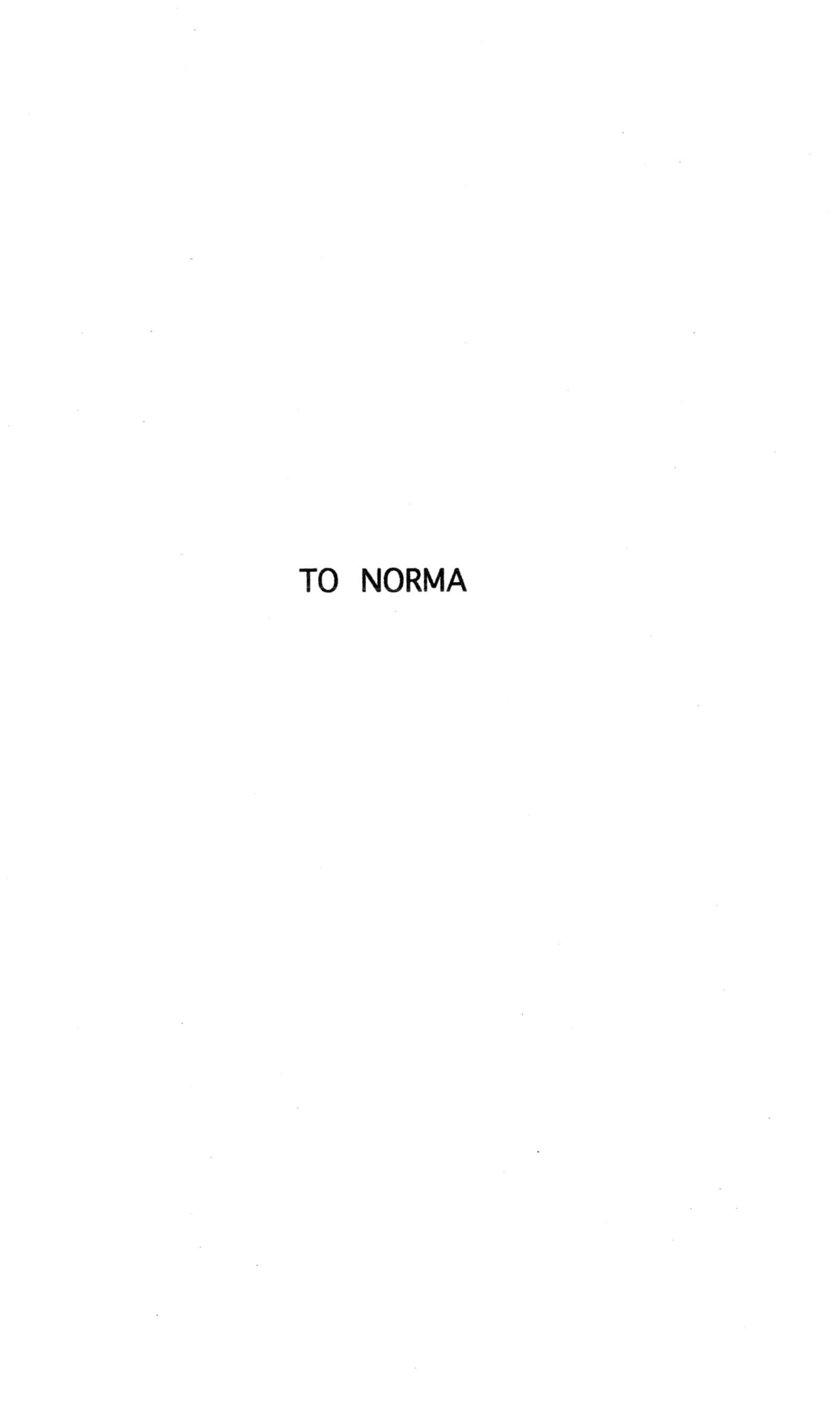

TO NORMA

ACKNOWLEDGMENTS

There is a sense of reverence in my gratitude to the patients who figure in these pages. I have been drawn to them with a need to know the worst of the world's pain, so that I might soothe it with whatever I have to offer. I have changed their names, but their real selves seem always to be looking over my shoulder, checking the details.

Unnamed are the people I have worked with, but they must know what the book owes to them: everything. I have been blessed to work side by side with men and women who not only share a social vision but know how to rely on one another in making it real.

I sigh when I think how far this book is from my first scrawled and scrambled words. The process has felt like a long and complicated gestation, with the final tumult of delivery coming long after the heyday of its engendering. Judy Kaplan was the guide, midwife, and minister to the words, the best editor a writer could hope for.

And my wife, Norma, merely makes everything possible and everything worthwhile.

INTRODUCTION

Imagine a group of people who are always together. They each work about 30 hours a week. Their labor is cooperative, proceeds at an easy pace, and is accompanied by pleasant chatter. There is a seamless connection between work, politics, homemaking, and play. Children are free to go anywhere, because everywhere they are watched, fed, and taught, as if every adult were a parent to every child. Talk is constant; a statement in one direction will be commented on from another. Conflicts are discussed until consensus is reached on what is best for everyone. There is no violence. When children fight, they are distracted by amusement or affection from an adult. People take only what they need, and what each needs is defined by what all need. There is only one privileged class: the children.

Is this a fantasy of utopian dreamers, or an idyll from a fictive Golden Age? Is it a vision of paradise?

Now imagine a group of people who have lost their humanity. They show no love, kindness, compassion, or caring. Sex is as perfunctory and about as joyful as defecation. Their only source of satisfaction is the misery of someone else. Children are abandoned by the age of three. The sick are beaten and robbed, the dead left unburied. There is no religion, no art, no hope, no rage, no sadness. There is only boredom, bitterness, envy, and suspicion.

Is this an existentialist's fable of doomed humanity? Is it a back ward of chronic paranoid psychotics? Or is it hell itself? No, these are, believe it or not, the same people separated by two generations.

The Mountain People is a book by the anthropologist Colin Turnbull that tells the story of the *Ik*, once a thriving tribe of hunter-gatherers who had lived in an organic relationship with one another and the land for as long as human history. Then, abruptly, the Ugandan government forced them to surrender their traditional lifestyle and remain on a reservation to "farm" in a single, isolated, desolate, drought-ridden region of countryside. The government would send "famine relief" when the tribe starved, but the tribe members who were sent for the food ate it all, forcing themselves to vomit so they could consume everything that was available.

Turnbull's story of the transformation of the *Ik* is a fragment in the progress of the world. It demonstrates what adversity can do to human behavior.

We are an adaptable species. This is our strength and hope, and it is also our tragedy. We can adapt to anything.

I remember my first revelation of the changes taking place in my hometown, New York City. I had took the train back from Boston a dozen or so years ago and having to use a bathroom, found my way to the men's room of Pennsylvania Station. I walked in and staggered a little at the sight of perhaps 20 men *living* there. One man was trying to bathe in the cold trickle at a sink. Another was building a fire in a corner to heat the remnants of some abandoned food. A third was curled at the base of a toilet, asleep. They hunkered or leaned or sat or sprawled in total silence.

Later as I wandered through streets which I had once thought scintillated with magic, I saw more and more of what I now know was only the beginning. I had known the underside of New York when I was growing up there, had seen the Bowery, dodged the pedophiles' grasps in the subway, heard the occasional howls of a lunatic or a drunk in the streets. But now it was endless and everywhere. And thereafter, each time I went back, I would experience with a new shock the quantum leap in the numbers of the homeless, the ratchet-turn of the wheels of decay.

And here, too, in Boston, once a "livable" city, what is inconceivable one day becomes mundane the next. We adapt. The questions for us are: What are the consequences of adaptation and to what do we *choose* to adapt?

The story of the *Ik* offers some understanding of how a certain kind of impoverishment results in an array of behaviors that can only be described as "sick." What do I mean by "impoverishment"? Certainly the *Ik* before their containment on a reservation were not wealthy. That is, in terms of income, the welfare benefits of a resident of Chelsea, Massachusetts, in 1992 would have seemed like a king's ransom to the tribe. And yet, in contrast to the life of the poor in Chelsea, there was a palpable richness to their lives as hunter-gatherers.

I am going to explore the nature of poverty in Chelsea, where I worked for 16 years as a psychiatrist at the Chelsea Community Counseling Center. I want to understand and make clear what it is about that kind of poverty that is pathogenic.

We tend to think of poverty as a matter of individuals, possibly of families, without resources, living below some "line" measured by experts in terms of income. But what can be seen with the *Ik* and what I saw in Chelsea is poverty as a social, shared, and interactional phenomenon.

Impoverishment in this sense is the dissolution of a gossamer network of reciprocal relationships, the loss of a sense of mutual accountability, the destruction of—let's call it—*community*.

We tend to think of mental illness as an aberration of individual behavior, a perturbation in one person's lifetime itinerary. It is usually described in terms of personal history and understood by many to reside at the synapses of neurons, if not within the very genes inside the nuclei of our cells.

We have lost our *common* sense about human behavior, not common as trivial or vulgar but as shared, a sense about ourselves *in common*. We have been trained to think of ourselves in a Newtonian billiard-ball universe in which relationships, if seen at all, are seen as the mere clicking of one impenetrable surface against another.

But when, as with the *Ik*, the invisible, ubiquitious network of relationships is actually ripped apart, there is as a consequence an array of behavior that could be judged as senseless, cruel, or mentally ill. With this perception of a tribe in decline, we may think of mental illness as the individual expression of what is socially experienced as poverty, and both poverty and mental illness as the manifestations of a *loss of community*.

Urban poverty is a whirlpool, a vortex of irresistible energy, a confluence of forces and events a little too large and a little too slow to be experienced as a war. But war it is, one in which we ourselves are both combatants and victims. In an ecological system, everything is connected and there is no Archimedean point from which to observe the devastation *out there*.

Poverty and mental illness in contemporary urban America can only be understood as a totality, but we have been carefully trained to perceive reality in segments, as if in snapshots through a cosmic zoom.

I will focus my camera on one community, a poor one in decline, and some individuals within it. I will relate the experience of individual distress, of *dis-ease*, that we call mental illness, to the nature of life in that community. I will tease apart particular constellations of forces within the whirlpool of poverty in which some of its vicious, implacable energy seems concentrated. Unemployment, compromised reproductive health, environmental pollution are pools of pathology, which together and when conjoined with currents of density, displacment, racism, malnutrition, crime, and child abuse, make up that whirlpool. And I find myself bobbing up and down within it, throwing a line here and there to someone who seems to be drowning. Occasionally I shout above the roar that *there* or *there* is the origin of some of this furious and destructive energy, a place where maybe it can be diverted or stopped.

I am, after all, a psychiatrist, a doctor. And if occasionally I observe and think like a social scientist collecting field notes, I also have a responsibility; I have taken a vow to try to reduce suffering. There are times when the instincts of the social scientist and the reflexes of the doctor come together, and new levels of understanding and possibilities of intervention are opened. It is such caesural moments, wedged within the raging prosody of the whirlpool, that I strive to capture in this book.

I remember one such moment in *The Mountain People*, a moment of such clarity and poignancy that to read it is to suddenly re-experience with an inner moan of longing and regret what it is to be human. It is a moment that strains and screams at the frontier of sanity and, in some way, helps establish it.

Turnbull noticed some activity near a ravine. An old woman, he discovered, had fallen in and been hurt. She was groaning in pain. At the edge of the ravine a group of young men watched and laughed. They were apparently prepared to spend the day entertained by the woman's agony and eventual death. As an anthropologist, a scientist, Turnbull's job was to watch the watchers, to record the scene. But he couldn't help throwing down his notes, climbing down into the ravine and carrying the woman on his back to her hut, accompanied by the mocking laughter of the onlookers.

Suddenly the old woman burst into tears and sobbed and moaned as if newly wracked with pain. Turnbull was alarmed that he might have dislocated a broken bone. But when he inquired, the old woman said that his kindness reminded her of what the life of the *Ik* had once been.

In this book I move back and forth across scales of magnitude in describing the relationship between poverty and mental illness, as if changing the objectives on a microscope or shifting the cosmic zoom.

After almost two decades in Chelsea I have come to know, at times to treat, the grandchildren of patients I saw when I first got there. (Children bear children in Chelsea.) One develops a sense of the intergenerational flow of pathology, with each encounter representing a moment in time as in a vast and endless river. My profession has come to believe that most of this pathology is hereditary, genetic. I will argue that despite the mythology of a classless and open society, despite the "little engine that could" that America is riding, it is poverty that is hereditary in Chelsea; people are trapped within it.

One mechanism of that trap has to do with reproductive health, involving a synergy of events and forces, each making the other more virulent, so that the net effect is greater than the sum of the component parts, a swirling vortex of destructive energy at the center of which is a fetus, a child soon to be born to the waiting midwives of poverty and mental illness. Teenage pregnancy, low birth weight, malnutrition, exposure to viruses, pollutants, drugs (legal as well as illegal), and other teratogens interact in Chelsea to foreclose the healthy development of children even before they are born.

The political economy of Chelsea is a mental health issue, not metaphorically but concretely and specifically. I once prepared an affidavit for a class action suit brought by the Coalition for the Homeless against the governor, my boss, which was quoted by the judge in his favorable (though ultimately ineffectual) decision. I was asked to demonstrate that homelessness causes mental illness rather than, as the conservatives argue, the other way around. Research, science, authority were used to state the obvious: when you take away a person's home you take away something of him- or herself.

Where does homelessness in Chelsea come from? I saw it happen. It does not come out of the blue. It is the consequence of real estate manipulations, of "gentrification," of greed. And I saw its horrifying, murderous, and almost routine connection with arson. I do not have the skill to treat the suffering of a mother of two children dead from a fire "of suspicious origin."

There is another array of suffering, which comes in the wake of yet another whirlpool within poverty: unemployment. Chelsea has the highest rate of unemployment in Massachusetts, which is among the highest in the nation. Not only does acute job loss predict a whole repertoire of bio-psycho-social distress (suicides, divorce, hypertension, peptic ulcers, strep infections, alcoholism, domestic violence, and so on) but chronic unemployment comes with its own particular burdens on the individual and the family. Brenner's massive studies on the relationship between unemployment and psychiatric hospitalization rates over the course of 127 years in the New York state hospital system are only a sample of a rich body of research about what happens when people cannot find work.

In a clinical setting, in traditional one-to-one psychiatric interchanges, to demonstrate to a middle-aged man that his sexual impotence is a symptom of unemployment is not easy. What techniques does one use to deal with the disease of unemployment?

This leads to a more general issue: how do our tools of psychotherapy and psychopharmacology work for the poor? *Do* they work?

I was trained in the psychoanalytic tradition, with that vocabulary and grammar, wearing that persona. It is brilliant, ingenious, revelatory, and almost completely irrelevant to the emotional lives of people in Chelsea. It was designed for more stable lives, ones distorted by lenses congealed in the past. Psychoanalytic psychotherapy is a heady, engrossing illumination of how the patterns of one's life fold and refold along lines that trip up the possibilities of satisfaction.

In Chelsea, the 50-minute hour of passive attention, of pushing toward the past, of highlighting the shards of unconscious material in free association, just does not work. Too much has happened since the last session. One cannot stop to adjust a watch in a whirlpool.

The poor are no less verbal than the middle class. Children who are thought to be wordless in the classroom chatter endlessly in the streets. There is a peculiar example of class and racial bias in the phenomenon of "alexithymia" invented by a couple of Boston psychoanalysts some years ago. It means the inability to express feelings in words, which is thought to be the major reason that poor people and minorities do not make good psychotherapy clients. Middle-class Americans are taught to say "I feel anxious" or "I am sad." Others, the rejected ones, *somatize.* And yet, who is to say where feelings reside? Does the statement "I feel sad" have more meaning than "My heart is breaking"? Is fear really more a mental construction than sweating and rapid pulse and hair rising at the back of the neck? The middle class lives in a world of words, so that not only art and music but even feelings must be translated into these dry, staccato symbols before they are thought to be real.

Nor are "they," the poor and those from the Third World, less curious about their emotional lives than others. A rural Puerto Rican may not have been socialized into thinking that *ataques* of pure anxiety and hysterical hallucinosis and fainting are caused by childhood trauma instead of a neighbor's hex. But all explanations are culturally determined, and all involve a basic curiosity about what one's emotional turmoil is connected to. Regardless of culture and class, all this complexity is capable of inquiry.

The poor are not less verbal or less curious than the rest of us, but the events of their lives have a different patterning. They occur rapidly and are endlessly toxic. One is forced to deal more with what happened yesterday than with what happened in one's childhood, though much happened then as well. Also, the assumption of much psychoanalytic treatment is that the unconscious somehow brings on the events of one's life, that we manipulate our own unhappiness. This may or may not be true in what is left of the middle class (I do not think it is generally true of its women), but it is certainly not true of the poor. People in Chelsea are, in fact, victimized and oppressed.

Psychoanalytic psychotherapy often focuses on the expression of suppressed or repressed emotions of hostility and sexuality. But life in Chelsea is marked by their all too free expression. Children are so habitually sexually abused that we take note with relief when we learn that one was not.

The expression of violence is constant and everywhere. Screaming arguments, physical fights, threats of murder, the routine carrying of weapons, and the tragically frequent resort to them, make for homes and streets that often resemble a war zone. Parties become gang wars as soon as they become boisterous, and the ethnic tensions among Anglos, Hispanics, and Southeast Asians present a constant threat of mass racial violence. Crack cocaine is everywhere, and the 56 bars in this small city of 1.8 square miles constantly generate a voluble and volatile presence of public drunkenness.

Despite Dr. Freud's ideas about consigned reservoirs of instinctual energy, to me it is obvious that anger does not become exhausted through its expression. It feeds on itself; the more it is expressed, the more it is experienced. Much of the psychotherapy of the poor in Chelsea has to be suppressive rather than expressive: resolving conflicts and helping people become less aggressive, teaching people how to wait and think before acting on a sexual impulse.

Perhaps oppression's worst feature is that the victims internalize the values of the oppressor. This is the terrible truth learned from survivors of concentration camps and torture, that victims all too often come to believe that they deserved their punishment.

The victims of poverty are taught to feel powerless. Jerome Kagan's studies of children in many cultural settings concluded that painfully early, by age six, lower-social-class children, in contrast to more affluent ones, have learned that what happens in their lives will never reflect their own initiative. Middle-class children are trained to feel that they can have some impact on the course of events. Poor children believe that external forces—luck, destiny, fate, or landlords—determine their lives. This is one reason there is so much gambling in Chelsea (the state lottery itself being a tax on the poor). Learned helplessness is a social phenomenon that results in impoverished mothers not believing they have the capacity to soothe an infant.

The apparent contradiction in the psychology of the victim of poverty who experiences both guilt (the feeling of having done something bad) and powerlessness (the feeling of being unable to do anything effective) is rarely articulated. As in a zen *koan*, when an apparently unresolvable dilemma is focused on, one may come to a reformulation of one's sense of self. The psychotherapy of the poor is most meaningful when it is directed at the conjoined powerlessness and self-blaming that characterize their emotional lives.

We all carry self-haters on our shoulders. Our thoughts about ourselves and our lives are always colored by shame (not having lived up to an expectation of ourselves) and guilt (having transgressed a limit). When a psychotherapist expresses concern and curiosity about a patient's life, he or she is saying, "Put your life into words for me." The very process is therapeutic because it may be the person's only opportunity in an entire lifetime to make a complete statement about him- or herself. Things put into words are less painful than fragments of unexpressed thought for the very reason that they are less contaminated by self-hatred.

The posture of the therapist is one of kind curiosity. "What happened?" we ask. "Why are you so unhappy?" "What are the patterns of your life?" "How did you get this way?" And, in a thousand different ways, "Who are you?" When a therapeutic alliance develops, the patient learns to identify with the kind curiosity of the therapist, and that very identification results in a maturation in the patient's ego. Instead of remaining stuck inside a state of rage or terror or longing, the patient can ask with that newly learned inner voice, "Why am I so angry or so frightened now?" or, "Why was I attracted to that bully?" A new sense of understanding and even control can emerge.

A kind and curious presence is a rare and precious element in the lives of the poor. It would be tragic if budgetary constraints, managed care proposals, or other business-minded managerial imperatives forever remove the prospects of psychotherapy for the poor and condemn them to case management and medication. Unfortunately, this is exactly what is happening today.

I find that with my commitment to community psychiatry and my conceptions of psychotherapy, I am at odds with the rest of my profession, with the psychiatric establishment. The whole nomenclature, the vocabulary of psychiatry and its diagnostic system, are irrelevant to my patients. (And, moreover, they confound the possibilities of thinking clearly.) The biogenetic "decade of the brain" mentality, with its arrogant assumptions, its inability to think contextually and, by the way, its thoughtless and sloppy science, leads systematically to a selective inattention to issues of ethnicity, social class, and other realities of life among the urban poor. I find I must challenge the presumptions and the methods and the very systems of classification that my profession has chosen as its institutional memory, its revealed truth, its ruling ideas.

The "scientist-psychiatrists" who define psychiatry in terms of neurotransmitters *do not know* the nature of mental illness in Chelsea any more than the psychopharmacologists know the extent to which their medications are abused and made into commodities on the streets.

While I use psychopharmacological agents, I never have the illusion that I am doing more than manipulating symptoms, brokering complaints, suppressing here, stimulating there, individuals' emotional experiences of forces that lie outside themselves, forces that are part of that furious whirlpool of urban poverty in which people thrash about, occasionally perishing, but often, miraculously, managing to survive.

The treatment of the impoverished mentally ill has always been a trickle-down affair. The trickle is now being shut off. With a sweep of his pen, a tax-conscious governor in Massachusetts ended my career in community psychiatry. At the very moment that I was trying to keep the embers of what was once a movement alive, I found myself pushed aside.

As more and more of us are flung into poverty, a psychiatry of poverty may one day be the only psychiatry left to practice. The poor are getting poorer and the middle class is losing ground; I cannot escape the painful conclusion that for much, perhaps most, of humanity the conditions of life are becoming like those of the *Ik*.

But that will not be the lingering image in the pages to come. A lot of what I portray in this book is desperately sad: brutalized children aging before one's eyes, women going from one battering relationship to another, men trapped within their own paranoia. My patients survive—not all, as we will see, but most survive. And the capacity to survive and, despite it all, to show humor, warmth, compassion, generativity, and hope is sustaining.

ONE

I recently found out that Robert, a former patient of mine, committed suicide by jumping from the fifth floor of his Chelsea apartment building. A reporter from the *Boston Globe* called to ask my opinion about his death: could it have been a consequence of the budget cuts that caused my departure from the clinic? She thought I had known about the suicide and became flustered and apologetic when she realized that I was learning about it from her.

It had been exactly a year since I had last seen him, when I had to tell him that after 15 years I could no longer be his psychiatrist. Along with 800 other state-employed mental health professionals who were working in outpatient clinics, I was being laid off.

I remember being reluctant to give him the reason he now had to go "across the bridge" to Boston to get his care at the Erich Lindemann Mental Health Center. Our sister clinic in nearby East Boston would have been more accessible, but was to be closed completely in a cost-cutting measure. And for "efficiency," our clinic, the Chelsea Community Counseling Center, now with only a third of its staff, was to become a privatized center for Spanish-speaking clients.

I knew Robert's racism only too well to mention that Puerto Rican and Central American people could continue using the clinic while he could not. He would learn it soon enough, however. Chelsea is a small town, and, in fact, Robert lived directly behind the clinic. The room in which the staff held its case conferences overlooked his apartment, and we occasionally, self-consciously, lowered the shades when we had a going-away party or a festive lunch that might include a bottle of champagne for a toast.

Alcohol was one of Robert's problems. He lived in a chronic paranoid state, suspicious of everyone, hyper-vigilant, quick to take offense. When he drank, his paranoia would blossom into wild and florid delusions of persecution involving the Mafia or the FBI.

Years ago, before I knew him, he had been hospitalized after being talked down from a roof in Boston. He had fled there, thinking, as in some ancient gangster movie or *sous-les-toits-de-Paris* spy flick or *King Kong* itself, that roofs were the avenue of escape from fictive pursuers. As the police climbed to the roof with that saccharine tone of voice they use with would-be jumpers, fantasy and reality began their slow terminal dance in his head. Deciding that he would rather die by his own hand than be tortured to death by imagined persecutors, he took a jagged piece of brick and began to slash at his abdomen and chest and wrist in a desperate, futile, final effort to be *in control.* He did little damage, and in tears of fear and rage, he was subdued, manacled, and sent to the inpatient unit of the Lindemann Center, where Stelazine and sobriety returned him to his usual level of paranoia.

He was left with a haunting, humiliating memory of the episode. After seeing me for ten years, he finally trusted me enough to describe it in such painful detail that suddenly, against his best effort, he broke down at the image of his wild, foresaken madness. "I'm sorry," he kept repeating. "It's all right," I kept responding.

He was otherwise a lonely and unsmiling man with a somber, forbidding look that periodically reddened into rage. He was in his fifties when we began our monthly visits. Divorced by his second wife who could no longer tolerate his jealous rages, he continued to follow her, showing up at the bars and drinking clubs that she frequented. She obtained a restraining order, and the judge ordered him to stay away from her. He said he had a "constitutional" right to go to the bar of his choice and claimed that she was actually pursuing *him* by being in places that he was likely to visit.

I said it is hard to lose someone you love, that it is hard to be rejected, that it is hard to be alone, but that we have to learn to accept loss—the usual litany of platitudes which paranoids rage against. Eventually he stopped following his ex-wife.

But he liked women and, until they got to know him better, they liked him. He had the rough, dog-faced good looks of a World War II vet. He liked to dance, and after a few drinks could even laugh a little. Middle-aged sexuality was free and easy in Chelsea before AIDS, and it was not unusual for a meeting at Bingo or a bar to end in bed before names were exchanged. But middle age after a career of heavy drinking was taking its toll on Robert, and impotence emerged as an intolerable burden. I counseled abstinence from both alcohol and sex for a while, but he quickly consulted a zealous urologist who inserted a human *os penis*, a prosthetic erection, a piece of plastic to offer the verisimilitude of passion. Robert gave his low-tech rejuvenation such a work-out, however, that his penis was injured when the rod perforated the *corporea cavernosa* and broke through the skin of his exhausted organ. "Never again," he said, and I helped him grieve the loss of youth.

He was frequently in fights, sometimes violent ones. Barrooms are not good places for paranoid people, and he was the kind of man who would respond to an accidental shove or slight with a challenge to step outside. At the Salvation Army Center, where a hot lunch cost 50 cents, he would loudly proclaim that other people were getting more meatballs or mashed potatoes than he was.

He had hypertension, a peptic ulcer, and coronary heart disease, all probably inevitable given his personality, but he also suffered from a vast variety of less specific aches and pains. As a hypochondriac with real diseases, he frequented a number of medical centers and outpatient clinics. He distrusted them all and often threatened them with malpractice suits. He was always carrying his x-rays from one to the other for a "second opinion." Several doctors refused to see him again.

Since I was the only one who ever really talked to him, he liked me. "You're the only doctor I can trust," he said. "Too bad you don't know anything about the body."

My "therapy" consisted of prescriptions for Stelazine along with my pedestrian advice and expressions of curiosity about his past. He had lots of stories about being exploited as a laborer, a "working stiff," when he did the dangerous work of installing fire escapes on the outsides of brick buildings. And he had lots of stories about the drinking and gold-bricking and fist-fighting he did in the army during the Second World War. He could never understand how we managed to win with soldiers like himself, but those days as "one of the boys" in the army were the happiest of his life.

As his reputation for paranoia spread, Robert was avoided by more and more of the lonely people in the bars and lunch centers and Bingo halls. He was becoming an isolated and cantankerous old man, and soon I was his major social contact. He never missed an appointment, and if I were late or out with an emergency, he complained bitterly to the receptionist, who had learned to wait out his abuse, after which he would apologize.

I told him the joke about the guy with the flat tire walking down a country road to a nearby house to borrow a jack. He so convinces himself that he will be refused that when the door opens to his knock he says, "You can keep your fucking jack." Robert laughed and said, "That's me, all right."

He raged against the government when he learned he had to travel to the Washington Street station of the MBTA in downtown Boston to get a reduced rate card. He said, "How the hell can they expect old and disabled people to go all the way to Boston to get what's due them?" I agreed and told him to write a letter to the *Boston Herald* about it. He said he couldn't. I helped him draft it. He rewrote it in his own handwriting and showed it to me with pride, but never sent it because he was afraid of retaliation. "They can print it without your name," I suggested. "I don't trust them," he said, but he kept the letter as a private trophy.

And then, after 15 years, I had to tell him that I could no longer be his doctor. He accepted this matter-of-factly and when I tried gently to touch on the sense of loss this might involve—perhaps something like losing a friend—he retreated to the brittle security of his pride and isolation. I suspected that he never would get to the clinic at Lindemann because of his feelings about the place and about Boston itself. But I also suspected that even if he got there, they would never be able to simulate this *thing* we had going, the propinquity, the ease, the casual wave across the street, this patient, enduring unprepossessing *therapy* of community mental health. At the Lindemann Center he would have been seen in a medication group and given a perfunctory greeting and his prescription by a tired and overworked nurse. And a year after I had last seen him, he climbed to the top floor of his building and jumped, his face clenched like a fist on the spike of anticipated pain, a moan of misery in his tightened throat, his body splayed against the rack of windows, including those of the clinic—windows he and I would never look through again.

Robert's death and my losses of clinic and career were not the only casualties of the state's budget cutting and privatization. I was told by a physician at the Massachusetts General Hospital that after the Chelsea clinic closed, a former clinic patient was seen in the Emergency Ward just about every day. Those endless ineffectual visits cost the taxpayers of

Massachusetts about $200 each. Robert was not the only patient we had managed to keep out of a psychiatric hospital. At incalculable cost, too many of our patients wound up in private "shock mills" or the psychiatric units of general hospitals, where over-priced "evaluations" were performed and the patients were discharged on the day their benefits expired.

With the closing of state hospitals, which followed the closing of state outpatient facilities, the private hospital with all its predatory financing and clinical ineffectuality is becoming the only resource for the mentally ill. It is a resource rarely granted to the most disorganized and needful people, the poor. The Massachusetts Department of Mental Health is calling this process not downsizing but "rightsizing," as if there were just too much fat in the system. They are attempting to replace the chronic wards of state hospitals with contracts to private companies who will develop "community residences."

Several such residences have existed for years in Chelsea. The clinic was often turned to by their overworked and poorly paid staffs. Without a community clinic, their residents will use the revolving doors of hospitals, which are rapidly closing to them. They will be "suspended" to the streets. The director of the Pine Street Inn, the largest shelter for the homeless in New England, announced that since privatization and the closing of the clinics, there has been a 40% increase in the number of severely mentally ill people at their door.

This did not come out of the blue. These are not random events or the idiosyncratic shrugs of reactionary public policy. They are the systematic effects of a collapsing economy.

I have lived through the rise and fall of the community mental health movement. It is as if I rode the last wave of a progressive system now ebbing on the shore. Beached, I am looking back.

A quarter of a century ago, I wrote a book about community psychiatry. I called it *The Absurd Healer*, not because I felt ridiculous, as I sometimes do now. Absurdity meant then that the possibilities of my work as a psychiatrist were endless, that its meaning might be found knurled in the center of meaninglessness itself, that purpose could creep up and tap one on the shoulder as long as one acted as if the words *struggle*, *idealism*, and *unity* were more than words.

But I was not alone. There was a movement. We had teachers, a literature, funding. I became involved, absorbed in the cultivation of this community garden. I took it seriously. And now, after what seems a very short time, I look up ready to ask for a hand from someone with more energy and youth and I find myself alone and the garden gone to seed. The teachers are dead or have given up the soil. The literature on mental health is in a foreign language, with words like *neurotransmitter* and *gene locus* and *diazepam receptor* on pages where one once read about power, poverty, and racism.

And the funding is gone. The government, for which I once worked, does not know me and cannot afford to support my labor.

The community mental health movement, which once stirred imagination and idealism like the civil rights movement, the War on Poverty, and eventually the peace and ecology movements, has become a dead leaf blown into a blind alley, its occasional rustle causing the merest sidelong glance from passersby busy with other things.

On occasion, however, when I describe community psychiatry to young professionals, I am impressed with the curiosity, the wonder at times, about a professional life so different from the purposes, values, and style in which they are now embedded. It may be a story worth telling.

One of the features of writing in one's advanced years is the sense of time in decades rather than years, which seem now too short and fleeting. I was socialized in the fifties, which, contrary to their TV image, were not the Golden Age. It was a time of brutality and deceit, and for many on the Left, a time of danger.

The Korean War was every bit as unjust as the one in Vietnam, but one could be called a traitor for questioning it. A malicious, alcoholic bully from Wisconsin was the most powerful political figure in the country. He mocked and terrorized intellectuals and clergy and union leaders and Jews. (There was no confusion in anyone's mind about who he meant by "atheistic communists.") Many jobs were lost, as well as some lives.

In my high school in Brooklyn, named after Abraham Lincoln, two teachers were summarily fired for having been communists in their youth. They were two of the most mild-mannered, non-political, and non-subversive teachers of math and English one could imagine. On the chance that they could poison our feckless brains (already protected from Russian H-bombs by the smelly, ink-stained, monogrammed desks under which we periodically hunkered), they were discharged without pay or benefits or the slightest objection from their union.

During my college years at Columbia University, communists were not permitted to speak on campus. On the other hand, an honorary degree was awarded to a fascist dictator named Castilio Armas who had with CIA assistance overthrown Guatemala's democratically elected Arbenz government, unleashing a half century of torment and torture.

In medical school at the University of Chicago, a few of us started a discussion group about the "social" aspects of medicine. We discussed the fact that if a resident of the adjacent Woodlawn ghetto were to collapse practically on the steps of the university's hospital, he or she would be transported by police ambulance seven miles away to Cook County Hospital. But other patients, almost always white, were flown in from thousands of miles away with such interesting and rare diseases as ulcerative colitis or systemic lupus. What did this mean to our medical education? (Later, as an intern at Boston City Hospital, I found I knew nothing about the everyday diseases devastating the lives of the poor.)

A junior member of the faculty pulled one of us aside in a friendly manner one day to let us know that certain members of the Department of Medicine were prepared to see someone suspended if such discussions continued. A word to the cowardly was sufficient. We were the Silent Generation; our tasks were to do our work, cultivate our careers, and keep our mouths shut.

Silence, ambition, and cowardice do not necessarily mean the absence of thought and feeling. Academia and medicine were the promised land. Whole generations of victims, refugees, and immigrants were meant to be redeemed by them. My extended family, barely rid of the stink of Ellis Island and the Lower East Side of New York, watched as if with bated breath while I, with my ordinary allotment of intelligence and perseverence, scratched at the golden gates of the promised city. They opened to me, and I could hear a swelling sigh of relief, gratitude, and pride behind me. Once inside, loping along with the rest of the elect, I found these grand places filled with lies, intimidation, and a refined kind of corruption. Much later did I learn how deep that went.

I turned to psychiatry in medical school as a place where I might discover some thoughtfulness and something like a social conscience. But contradictions could be found there as well. In the fifties, psychiatry was a bi-modal affair. At the top was a thin veneer of psychoanalytic sophistication. Beneath it was a swollen mass of 50,000 impoverished human beings forgotten on the back wards of state hospitals.

Psychoanalysis was a European affair, coming to this country with refugees from Hitler. The bearded, accented analyst behind the couch came to be the cultural archetype of psychiatry, despite the fact that analysis was available only to a small segment of upper-class Americans, while for most psychiatric patients the state hospital was all there was.

Grafted onto American stock, psychoanalysis blossomed into something new and different. It had originally been an intellectual and scholarly pursuit, more an instrument for understanding history and society than for treating its unhappy and dysfunctional members. As part of the European intellectual tradition, psychoanalytic thinking shared common ground with Marxism; many of its practitioners, including those closest to Sigmund Freud, were, in fact, Marxists.

But refugee status can have a remarkably conservatizing effect. Having been quickly adopted by an individualistic and competitive culture, enriched by an upper-class clientele, and possessed with the status of tenured professorships, psychoanalysts in America conveniently forgot their common ground with Marxist thinking.

At the other antipode of psychiatry were the overcrowded, dehumanized institutions which had been designed to be progressive a century before. Dorothea Dix had been shocked at the sight of the mentally ill in the streets, jails, and "almshouses" (the homeless shelters of the era). Going from state to state, she was able to convince ordinarily economy-minded legislatures (not known for their responsiveness to female reformers) to appropriate relatively large amounts of money for the construction of a state hospital system. The classic Kirkbride building designs, now seen as grotesquely dated, were then the most advanced conception of psychiatric architecture. The land chosen for their sites was among the most fertile and beautiful available. To this day, these depressing buildings can be found on landscaped parks rolling gently down to lakes or cradled within pristine forests.

Shortly before she died, Ms. Dix had the opportunity to visit the state hospitals built under her influence. She became increasingly embittered and depressed at the spectre of degraded human beings stored away and forgotten rather than residing in hopeful centers of rehabilitation.

What went wrong? As the nineteenth century came to a close, the world was caught up in one of its cycles of economic depression. American cities became crowded with displaced, impoverished European immigrants. Attitudes toward the mentally ill shifted from compassion to control, as the new patients came to include culturally different and economically threatening people, who were called "the foreign pauper insane."

And psychiatric practice, perhaps the most sensitive indicator of the prevailing social system, changed its focus from a social rehabilitation orientation to a biological and medically dominated one. The discovery that the syphilis spirochete caused a form of insanity provided the scientific baptism for an ideology that defined medical research and pharmacological treatment as the only rational approach to the mentally ill.

And now, to close the historical circle, during yet another *fin de siècle* period of economic decline, with the remnants of the community mental health movement being stamped out, with the states closing mental hospitals and the streets crowded with the homeless mentally ill, with psychiatrists repudiating both compassion and rehabilitation in a rigid mindset of biological determinism, we are returning to a situation that Dorothea Dix found unacceptable over a century ago.

As the fifties ground on, another development in psychiatry emerged. Tranquilizers they were called unapologetically, and tranquilizers they were. And so they remain, though by now the profession has been carefully trained by the pharmaceutical industry to call them "anti-psychotics" and "anxiolytics."

The emergence of the "major" tranquilizers, including Thorazine and Stelazine, was dramatic. They were reported to bring about sudden cures in people who were hopelessly psychotic; the straight jackets and padded cells for violent patients were soon replaced by injections or little M&M-like pills. This was described as a "revolution," giving the word a new and respectable meaning.

It took a few years for the profession to learn about the downside of tranquilizers, the "side effects," as they are called, as if merely the penumbral splatter of magic bullets. Too often doctors felt that unless patients were made zombie-like from muscle stiffness, tremors, and a mask-of-death expression, they were not getting the full therapeutic effect from the drug. It was several decades before we learned that some side effects do not go away when the drug is stopped. Thousands of patients have a permanent legacy of facial twitching and gesticulating called "tardive dyskinesia." Others have died from peculiar syndromes of fever and muscle spasms or acute blood reactions.

Sophisticated, multi-hospital studies of the effects of the major tranquilizers have concluded that while they were useful in controlling agitation and the potential for violence, as well as the intensity of hallucinations and delusions (so-called "positive" symptoms), they were useless in controlling—and possibly even exacerbated—the "negative" symptoms of social withdrawal and passivity. They worked well for acutely psychotic patients (as did many other things, such as sedatives and time itself), but for chronic patients who make up most of the hospitalized population, they functioned primarily as chemical restraints.

The "minor" tranquilizers, or anti-anxiety drugs, were the fellow travelers of the pharmacological revolution. They are basically sedatives in that you take a little to feel relaxed and a little bit more to go to sleep. The chemicals being used shifted from the barbiturates to non-barbiturate sedatives like Doriden to the meprobamates like Equanil or Miltown (named for the town in New Jersey where they were made). At the final stage of maturation were the benzodiazepines such as Librium, Valium, Halcion, Serax, Tranxene, and Xanax, which differ only in terms of their duration of action.

The shifting tides of popularity in psychiatric drugs have nothing to do with pharmacological rationality, but rather with the rhythms of patent expiration and the power of medical advertisements—in other words, profits.

Valium was until recently the most popular anodyne in the history of the world not because of its superiority to Librium (which it resembles closely) but because of a woman named Jan. She was the best-known patient in America, gracing the center and endpages of almost every medical publication for years. The ad consisted of a series of snapshots throughout her fictive life. She was seen first as a little girl at her own birthday party, her father leaning over her head a little too closely. Later she is at her prom pulling away with a frown from her beamingly pubescent date. Later still she is pulling away from the macho advances of the T-shirted owner of a Chevy Nova. The final picture shows her looking prim and sad on the deck of a ship headed for Europe. The copy reads that "the Purser had to take this photo because she was traveling alone." It goes on to remind us that we "have all seen patients like Jan," and suggests that Valium can be helpful for the problem, which by now everybody knows to be her fear of sex. The patent on Valium has since run out, but the Roche company simply redesigned their unprepossessing tablet, adding a sculptural V-shaped hole, which they then patented. This was associated with a major media blitz directed at both physicians and the public about the (much exaggerated) risks of generic drugs.

In any case, Xanax (which is still under patent) is now the hot item on the benzodiazepine market and has replaced Valium as a street drug as well. The fifties were called "the age of anxiety." Little did we know.

TWO

The sixties came in like a breath of fresh air. Youth defined the decade. The baby boomers hit their teens and the Ikes and Adenauers of the world were replaced by Kennedy, Brandt, and Fidel. On the radio, out of a desert of "bubble-gum" rock, were heard the Beatles with sounds and words as subtle, complex, and *relevant* as they were accessible. The word *revolution* became a commonplace, and social justice became the standard against which all issues were measured.

On college campuses, the generation that silently endured McCarthyism was blown aside by students who went to the South to march for civil rights, who challenged the vested interests of their own universities, and who cheered the image of Lenin at the movies. The decade was darkened by the assassinations of the Kennedys and King and the war in Vietnam, which grew to be America's definition in the world and the rallying point for the New Left.

While my personal consciousness of the world was forged in the fifties, it was during the sixties that I developed a professional identity compatible with a social purpose. But it came slowly.

I graduated from the University of Chicago School of Medicine in 1961. By that time I had decided that psychiatrists were the most intelligent of all physicians, the ones asking the interesting questions. They went beyond "What is the diagnosis?" and "What is the treatment?" (the latter answered differently depending on whether one were on a medical or a surgical floor) and asked, "Why did this person become sick at this time?" and even, "What does it mean to be sick?"

I had come from a pre-medical education in philosophy, and hungered for an inquiring and kind conception of medicine in the midst of a mine field of facts and techniques. In medical school, students were made to feel tense and insecure, like marine recruits before a whole battalion of drill instructors. We were constantly subject to humiliation, comforted only by the fantastic hope that someday we too could humiliate others. Psychiatrists, however, in contrast to the other specialists, tended to be *more* respectful of their students as well as of their patients. They seemed to feel that only in an atmosphere of mutual respect was it possible to *learn* from a patient what he or she was suffering. The stellar surgeons and internists tended to be more charismatic, with their piercing eyes and dexterous hands and magical sniffing out of esoteric diagnoses. There was something more level and sensible about the psychiatrists, and at the same time, more profound. I became attached to them, going on their rounds, participating in research activities, and eventually I came to be "their" student.

One day they were visited by a British psychiatrist named Maxwell Jones. He had developed an innovative program for World War II veterans suffering from what was called "effort syndrome," a kind of malignant hypochondriasis and incapacity to perform any work. The program consisted of residence in a facility dominated by Jones himself, but in the daily control of pragmatically trained, nonprofessional "social therapists," who ministered in an environment of endless group therapy, relentless confrontation, and reciprocal responsibilities. The hierarchies between staff and patients were reduced to a minimum, and decision making was participatory, with privileges and discharges decided by the entire "community."

I listened hungrily as he described a "sense of community" as itself therapeutic. He went on to describe a town in Belgium he had just visited where mental patients were housed in the homes of peasants. The entire ambience of the community revolved around incorporating the mentally ill into the fabric of its daily life. It was named Gheel, or Geel in its Flemish version. In 1959, I spent three months in Geel observing its day-to-day activities and doing what turned out to be the first research ever done there. My study compared the families who had dropped out of the program with those who continued to host patients in their homes. It touched on the legendary origins of the place, the economy of small farms, and the emerging influences of industrialization and urbanization, which I learned were beginning to erode the tradition of the community.

The report attracted attention, describing an experiment that sounded modern but was actually ancient, as many good ideas turn out to be. It fit in with the movement toward a noninstitutional approach to the care of the chronically ill, a movement that was soon to take on a whole new meaning when the term "deinstitutionalization" emerged as a distortion of community mental health.

The experience acted as a fixative on my career as a community psychiatrist. A medical internship at Boston City Hospital was a rite of passage, a place to learn about medicine and the poor and the limits of my own capacities. Even then, exhausted as I was after taking a history and doing a physical exam and writing orders, I could not resist asking, "How are things at home?" I began to learn a little of the endless complexity in the lives of the poor and how their illnesses grew from and added to that complexity.

In 1962, I started a psychiatric residency at Massachusetts General Hospital, where I came under the influence of Erich Lindemann. I also became a commissioned officer in the United States Public Health Service as a Fellow of the Mental Health Career Development Program.

During the Kennedy administration, there was not only a national commitment to do something about the plight of the mentally ill, but also a period of economic prosperity that made it possible. Everybody drove American cars, the dollar ruled the world, and there were jobs. The war in Vietnam and the crazy-quilt inflation that came with it had not yet emerged as the commanding presence in American policy. Domestic programs were designed with a "damn the cost" mentality that had never before and will probably never again be seen.

The Community Mental Health Services Act of 1963 was passed in two fragmented versions because the American Medical Association, in its terror of "socialized medicine," was opposed to the idea of federal money being used to pay the salaries of physicians and other workers in a mental health setting. It was more than a year before other lobbying efforts, including those of the American Psychiatric Association (who were, after all, physicians, too), caught up with them, and staffing grants were finally enacted.

The legislation was in most respects rather tepid and conventional. Money was channeled through the states to build and staff community mental health centers, which were obliged to provide the usual array of services—inpatient, outpatient, day hospital, emergency, and consultation. The legislation was progressive in that the financial structure was not based on a user-insurance system but on program support. The costs of providing whatever services deemed appropriate for a particular community were to be entirely underwritten by the government. This differed from the Medicare system, also enacted at that time, which was essentially a universal health insurance program for the elderly and disabled built into the Social Security laws. Some health planners had predicted that by expanding the consumership of a commodity that remains in private, essentially monopolistic hands, and not at the same time extending the *production* and *distribution* of health care services, the result will be an increase in its price. With the enactment of Title 18 of the Social Security Amendments, the hospital where I was working increased its fees for an outpatient visit from $15 to $60 and its inpatient rates comparably. The treatment was the same, but many hospitals and doctors got rich on Medicare, and it remains an argument whether or not health care for the impoverished elderly actually improved.

The community mental health center legislation was designed not only to develop a whole new array of resources in health care, but to provide a model for a universal, egalitarian, and non-class-ridden system of care. Another progressive feature of the law was that it was population-based. A community was defined, somewhat arbitrarily, as 75,000 to 200,000 people living contiguously. The mental health needs of each community were to be addressed in a grant application consistent with a statewide comprehensive plan. These plans as drafted did not always represent the epitome of social-psychiatric sophistication. One "comprehensive" plan from a state in the South was sent to NIMH in pencil. But it was, at least in theory, possible for the designers of a community program to think about and attempt to address every facet of mental health in that community, such as race relations, the closing of an industrial plant, urban renewal, poverty itself. This was rarely done in actuality, but programs designed by some communities revealed a commitment to primary prevention and social change. Progressive politics and community psychiatry could conceivably find themselves on the same path.

Obviously, the "manpower" (as it was called) for these programs had to be developed, as there were limited numbers of mental health professionals already in practice and few of those were inclined to give up lucrative private practices in exchange for a publicly funded salaried position. Special grants encouraged general practitioners to go into psychiatry. Specialized postgraduate programs in community psychiatry were established. I was among the first to enlist in the elite Mental Health Career Development Fellow Program.

Money was no object. The story in circulation was that the director of NIMH, Dr. Robert Felix, was asked for his administratively approved budget at the annual meeting of the House Appropriations Committee. When this had been read, the committee chair then asked Dr. Felix what a "dream" budget might look like. This alternative budget, by informal agreement, was pulled out, read, and ultimately authorized. NIMH, which started out as just one of the Institutes of Health, soon had a budget equal to all the others combined and before long was made a separate agency. Interestingly, at the same time that hundreds of millions of dollars were appropriated each year to develop community mental health centers as alternatives to the state hospital system, NIMH was also making millions available to those very hospitals. It was not anticipated that state hospitals would close their doors until they were rendered useless by a functional community alternative, if ever.

"Deinstitutionalization" and its unhappy consequences were *not* part of the community mental health legislation or movement. That came later when the money ran out. Deinstitutionalization became a method for states to cut their mental health budgets by closing wards or whole hospitals and sending chronic patients into the streets with politically palatable rationalizations of community mental health jargon.

Social programs do not function in an economic vacuum. They always represent a "trickle down" of the wealth in a capitalist society. When surplus capital begins to dwindle, the rhetoric of social welfare remains without the substance, a grotesque pseudomorph of concern. This provides a soothing balm to the conscience of liberals and functions as a form of social control. But I am running ahead of the decade.

NIMH made a major investment in mental health research during the sixties. However, unlike the "war on cancer" or "cure for schizophrenia" variety of research that dominates the current scene, federally supported research was, consistent with the times, socially meaningful. Much of the research focused on epidemiology but not, as today, in terms of specific diagnostic categories. Investigators looked at incidents of illness or hospitalization or objectively defined measures of global incapacity (*dis-ease* or *dys-function*) that could relate the extent of mental disability in the entire community to such issues as unemployment, social density, migration, minority status, and poverty. It was not automatically assumed, as it is now, that there are specific disease categories of mental illness, each with their own specific etiologies, courses, and treatments. Instead, consonant with public health thinking, dynamic relationships between social forces and individual pathology were explored. This kind of research, in the hands of people like Hollingshead and Redlich, Pasamanick, Leighton, and Srole, determined persuasively that however mental illness is defined and however social class is measured, the lower the social class, the higher the incidence and severity of mental illness.

One of the studies supported by NIMH was under the direction of Erich Lindemann, my teacher at Massachusetts General Hospital. He introduced himself and his work to us with a gesture in the direction of the West End community of Boston just outside the windows of the Bulfinch building where we were sitting. It was 1962 and the West End was in the process of being destroyed in one of the earliest and most improvident urban renewal programs. It was a heterogeneous, working-class community with a special coherence and identity, whose residents called themselves "Westenders" rather than Bostonians. It was widely considered one of the best neighborhoods in America: vigorous, pluralistic, proud, and safe because of the many "eyes on the street." It was completely destroyed to make way for the usual wrack of enterprise, including shopping centers, high-rise, upper-middle-class apartment houses, a Holiday Inn, and some government buildings, among which was to appear the Erich Lindemann Mental Health Center. A decade later, this structure was to become a cruel and ironic memorial to a man with a very different conception of mental health.

In the sixties, Lindemann was interested in the effects on Westenders of the destruction of their community. He hypothesized that apart from the stress of moving, there would be a specific assault to their emotional welfare as a result of the loss of their community. In fact, it was later determined that the psychiatric incidence rate (the number of people becoming ill enough to require treatment) *doubled* among those relocated from the West End.

Think how far we have come. A few years ago, Mayor Koch addressed a meeting of the American Psychological Association in New York. He received a standing ovation after describing the extent of mental illness among the homeless of the city, describing people so dysfunctional that they soiled themselves. There is just no point in providing housing for such people, he argued. They need to be "treated," to be put away.

New York City had systematically destroyed its low-income housing. Tax abatements were given to wealthy developers who "rehabilitated" apartment houses so that upper-class condos could replace the tenements of the poor. Single-room-occupancy hotels and rooming houses disappeared—places where the impoverished and alienated of the city could have their own place to sleep and be sheltered from the icy winds that swirl through the high-rise canyons of Manhattan. The poor were forced onto the dimly lit extensions of subway platforms, into cardboard boxes under highways, or into cavernous armories where rape and robbery were the cost of a cot. And after this, the mayor of this great city and the representatives of America's mental health professionals agreed with enthusiasm that giving homes to such people is a waste of time and money.

Thirty years ago, in a different era, Lindemann proved that it was a cruel devastation of people's mental health to be relocated from one community to already existing homes in another. His finger pointing in a *j'accuse* gesture at the wrecking machines outside the window, Lindemann said, "It is a fiction that mental illness resides within the individual." One does not hear such things now from professors of psychiatry. It was not all that common in the sixties, either. Lindemann, in his quiet, avuncular, somewhat disorganized way, was a revolutionary without a revolution. He had originally studied philosophy and came to psychiatry and psychoanalysis through neurology, not unlike Freud. He had been the "fair-haired boy" of the Boston Psychoanalytic Society and was slated to be its leader until he began talking about "the community." He was soon considered a renegade.

Lindemann had established an international reputation through his studies of grief among the survivors of the Coconut Grove fire, a famous nightclub disaster in which dozens of people burned to death. He observed and analyzed the nature of grief as a normal rather than pathological process. From him, I learned about the arbitrary and specious boundaries between illness and health and between the individual and society.

Most of the rest of psychiatric education at the time revolved around traditional psychoanalytic dogma. It was not lost upon trainees in psychiatry that virtually all of its leaders and tastemakers were analysts, and that the princes of the profession were the senior and training analysts of the local psychoanalytic institute.

Community psychiatry incorporated an ideology that was at odds with the elitism of psychoanalysis. It recognized the need for "indigenous" nonprofessional mental health workers, particularly in ethnic minority communities. It also, though rather perfunctorily, accepted the idea of community participation in the direction of mental health programs. This borrowed from, but rarely went as far as, the anti-poverty legislation of the time, which incorporated the concept of "maximum feasible participation of the poor." (For the first time in history, the recipients of a welfare program could have something to say about its design and implementation.) But in mental health, in such places as the South Bronx, Philadelphia, and Roxbury, Massachusetts, when moves were made in the direction of community control, conflict arose between community boards and medical staffs, who were unaccustomed to being challenged (or even questioned) about their judgments in professional matters. In a few dramatic instances, radical professionals, allied with nonprofessionals and community board members, organized protests, sit-ins, or strikes.

Toward the end of my training in psychiatry, one of my teachers, a traditional psychoanalyst, asked me if I still intended to pursue a career in community psychiatry. When I said, "Yes, more than ever," he confided that he and his colleagues had originally thought of me as "analytic material," but that my insistence on a career line so at odds with theirs suggested deeper problems. He recommended that I go into therapy to try to overcome these clearly neurotic tendencies.

I left the Massachusetts General Hospital the same year as Erich Lindemann. Harvard retired him at 65. He did not share my optimism about community mental health legislation; he doubted that much could come from an enterprise so firmly in the hands of our profession.

Ironically, years later, as his "star" pupil, I was asked to introduce the bill in the state legislature to give his name to the Erich Lindemann Mental Health Center, an architectural monstrosity built in the West End, where children once skipped rope and women called from windows as they hung laundry on fire escapes, where men chattered in front of barber shops and people who were Polish, Irish, and Italian treated each other as neighbors.

The year I spent at Harvard at the Laboratory of Community Psychiatry as a fellow was the closest I ever came to a purely academic experience. Even my undergraduate years were burdened with part-time jobs and a long subway commute from Brooklyn to Morningside Heights in Manhattan. But for a year at Harvard, I did nothing but read, attend seminars, learn about mental health consultation, and do some research. Since then, I have always seen the academic environment as an Elysian Field of scholarly self-indulgence, something not to be taken too seriously.

But I took advantage of it. During the summer, I arranged to do field work in California, studying the linkages among service agencies in Contra Costa County. I was involved in a "Design Fete" in Houston, in which architects, planners, social scientists, and mental health professionals designed prototypical mental health centers for various physical and social environments. In addition, I consulted on a regular basis with the Visiting Nurse Association and the Massachusetts Rehabilitation Commission. And I did some research, in a barroom.

I was curious about the putative role of the bartender as a psychotherapist. Cocktail lounge bartenders are too busy to talk to people, I discovered from discussions with the bartenders' union, but in local taverns, particularly ones with a stable and regular clientele, the bartender often functions as a group therapist of sorts. I did a "participant-observer" study in a tavern in Charlestown, a working-class community soon to be devastated by gentrification. The clientele resided for the most part in rooming houses and used the barroom as their salon.

The experience gave me a renewed respect for the spontaneous systems of mutual support, the natural "caretakers" as Lindemann called them, which any collective of humans seems capable of forming. If there is any single theme that runs through and dominates the entire course of community mental health and social psychiatry, it is that community mental health *is* mutual support and the best any professional can do is to ally with it.

As part of my training in sociology and community dynamics, I began to spend time with the staff of the NAACP in Roxbury. My official purpose was to help them identify complaints which might be more "paranoid" than based in reality, but I was not particularly helpful, as most of the people in their community lived a daily life of paranoid reality. I began to appreciate how endless were the costs of being black in urban American and the extent to which the color line, compounded with poverty, was the deepest and most devastating fault in American society.

One day in the NAACP office, between sounds of rhythm and blues beating from the "soul station," WILD, a curious message was suddenly broadcast. It announced a special healing service that was to be performed at the Miracle Temple for men who had been "fixed." The service was to be rendered by "that young man of miracles," Reverend Ike, who guaranteed to "remove the fix."

I turned to one of the secretaries and asked her what it meant. She giggled and changed the subject. When I persisted, she finally revealed that men in the community who had trouble sustaining an erection would say a "fix" had been put on them. Reverend Ike claimed to rid them of it.

Sexual impotence is a notoriously fickle and emotionally based condition, and I assumed that Reverend Ike was providing a mental health service for many men who would not dream of consulting a psychiatrist. I decided to try to meet the young man of miracle. It was not easy. No phone number was listed for the Miracle Temple, and the radio station would not give me his home address. When I spoke with the manager of the station, he explained that so many people called wanting Ike's services that they had to protect him from being overwhelmed. When I explained my purpose, he became interested and later called back, reporting with some enthusiasm that Reverend Ike would be delighted to meet me. They had apparently shared a laugh over the interest of a shrink from Harvard. But before he gave me the coveted number, he asked how I would feel about being on the radio with Ike, on a public service program called "Action 1090." Something like "Religion vs. Psychiatry for the Ghetto" was what he had in mind. I was not too happy about the debate format, but was up for anything in those days. Ike had already agreed to do it, happy for some free radio time.

Frederick Eikerenkoetter, better known and more easily spelled as Reverend Ike, was as amiable on the phone as on the radio. He suggested that we meet for lunch at Jimmy's Harborside, a sprawling, glitzy seafood establishment. He made a conspicuous entrance in a long Lincoln with a built-in TV. (This was before the era of stretch limos.) He was a man of my age exactly, but with his silk suit, diamond-and-gold jewelry, and his hair slicked back to a French roll, he cut a far more dramatic figure than my gray Ivy-League self. When he went to the bathroom, the hostess asked me in a hushed whisper, "Isn't he a famous actor or something?" He looked as if he should have been. A man as energetic and articulate as he was handsome, he had a natural inclination to be in the center of things. Our radio enterprise grew to be a mini-series, with several weekly encounters well advertised by the station. I considered it a triumph that toward the end, the program came to be called "Religion *and* Psychiatry for the Ghetto."

We became friends. There was a peculiar complementarity in two healers with big mouths, each playing the other for all he was worth. I invited him to Harvard, where he charmed a room full of jaded psychiatrists, and he invited me to a healing service at the Miracle Temple. This, despite the hieratic name, was an unprepossessing brownstone in the South End to which several dozen men and women came on a Sunday afternoon.

I declined a warm invitation to share the podium with Reverend Ike. It was a three-hour service with music provided by the organist (his wife, who was also the treasurer of the church), a choir of a dozen spirited women in crimson robes, with Ike's strong baritone voice blending in and overcoming the singing and clapping of the choir and congregation. He talked constantly through and around the music, a smooth, seamless, inspirational patter of hope and humor.

"Let's hear a hand for the Lord," he suddenly shouted, interrupting himself in response to some indefinable signal that the energy level in the room had dipped. There was a response of lively applause.

"That sounds like a hand for a politician. I said a hand for *THE LORD!*" And the room exploded into a happy, cheering, exuberant ovation.

The only moralizing in his message was his expression of contempt for competing storefront ministers in the community who, he declared, announced "numbers" for the illegal lottery system that provided some of the substructural economy of the ghetto.

The healing part of the service was its climax. As the music and the patter rose in pitch, there were spontaneous shouts of "I love you, Jesus" and "I hear you, Lord" and "Yes! YES!" after every hortatory phrase from the minister. At one point, with a scream, a woman fell to the floor in the aisle that ran down the center of the rows of brown folding chairs. I restrained an impulse to attend to her in the useless way doctors have during an epileptic seizure. Without stopping his singing, Ike stepped from the podium and touched her forehead with his index finger. The rings on his hand shimmered. She jumped as if shocked and went back to her seat.

Ike called up to the front a few people, who in brief phrases described how a healing cloth blessed by Ike had cured one or another ailment—an arthritic knee, an asthma attack, seizures. I saw no miracles before my eyes, and with each testimonial to the "prayer cloth," Ike abjured the survivor to be sure he or she checked with a physician to be certain that the illness was indeed gone. The only skepticism in the room was in my small corner.

No money was collected at the meeting. The services were taped and broadcast on radio stations all over the world during time purchased at commercial rates by the church. At the end of each tape, Ike's voice urged listeners to send for their "absolutely free" prayer cloth, which was personally blessed by him. "The blessings of The Lord are free," he added, "but the costs of our ministry are great." The radio faithful, it was suggested, would get additional benefit attendant upon their concern for these costs.

Later, Ike showed me the bolts of red material from which the two-inch square prayer cloths were sheared, later to be placed on the affected parts of the bodies of thousands of listeners. He never told me how much money was collected, but in an aside, he bemoaned the $5,000 per *month* cost of the material itself.

He also showed me examples of the stacks of letters that came with contributions or requests for additional prayer cloths. One after another chosen at random revealed enthusiastic acclaim or reports of cures. Occasionally, the letters were tinged with an erotic element and, rarely, though often enough for him to feel the need for an armed chauffeur, there was an angry threat from the husband or boyfriend of a congregant whose feelings about the minister involved a confusion of passions.

One night as we were drinking some of his expensive brandy, I asked him how he really felt about what he was doing. I half expected a complicitous wink or a little smile, but after a pause, he said with seriousness, "I don't know, Matt. You saw those letters. . . ." He looked down. "Something is coming through these hands."

I took that at face value as the statement of a man a little astonished at finding himself the agent of forces more powerful and mysterious than he himself had thought possible. However, as the years went on, the something else that was coming through his hands began to influence his preaching more directly. His ministry changed in the seventies from a focus on healing to something straightforwardly mercenary. He stopped speaking about prayer cloths or the Lord's cures and preached about money.

It was, I suppose, the most honest expression of a certain perennial variety of piety, praying for wealth. He did not give out "numbers," but he now paraded before the devout person after person whose five-, ten-, or twenty-dollar bills sent to Ike's church had been personally blessed by him so that hundreds or thousands of dollars rained in upon the believer. Ike was now blessing money itself. His message began to approach a social commentary for the first time: "The lack of money is the root of all evil."

The IRS agreed and attempted to sue him for back taxes. Their argument was that his lifestyle was inconsistent with that of a man of the cloth. Ike's lawyers argued that the same position would have to be taken toward the Roman Catholic Church, with particular reference to the Fifth Avenue residence of the Cardinal of New York. The suit was apparently dropped.

I have lost contact with Revered Ike, but I think about him from time to time. I have no idea what impact my relationship with him had on my development as a community psychiatrist, but "something" was "coming through."

THREE

In 1966, I went to work for the federal government, the employer of last resort. I became the staff psychiatrist, and before long was the Acting Chief, of the Metro Center, a branch of the National Institute of Mental Health established with a multimillion-dollar budget to do something about the mental health of cities.

We worked closely with the Office of Economic Opportunity (OEO), the Justice Department, the Department of Housing and Urban Development, and the Kerner Commission on Urban Violence to find out why cities had riots. Anyone with an ounce of understanding about racism and poverty could answer the question, but the government needs to pay for "studies" before it chooses to ignore a social problem.

So I became an expert on cities, quickly learning the language of social science research, city planning, and urban politics. Most of what I spoke about was a rehash of lib-rad sentimentality, but I wore the mantle of authority, so whatever I had to say about race relations, power, and poverty was quoted in the press and on television.

In contrast to the fatigued and despairing response to the L.A. riots of 1992, which occured at a time of economic decline, in the sixties confidence was still in the air. It is hard to think and write clearly about that period from the disadvantaged viewpoint of this one. The country, the whole world, it seemed, was in a paroxysm of hope. Prague and Paris and even Rome percolated with the same expectations of change as Detroit and Newark. The participants in the street riots were not, we found, the most recent migrants from the South, those who were the most oppressed, impoverished, and desperate residents of the ghettos. They tended to be second- or third-generation migrants, already urbanized, and to a large extent, already employed. It was their frustrated expectations for a more secure and comfortable existence that fed the violence—the irritations of hope, not the paralysis of despair.

This insight was later to be picked up by such manipulative reactionaries as Daniel Patrick Moynihan, who, as advisor to Richard Nixon, urged a policy of "benign neglect" toward the cities, the black, and the poor. What he meant was that when people are more beaten down, exploited, and miserable, they become less troublesome. This was soon to become the guiding principle of U.S. domestic policy.

But in the sixties, there was a real conviction that even here, "in the belly of the beast," social change could take place. Popular music spoke to its youthful listeners about change. Every profession, professionalism itself, was seen by its most vigorous practitioners as an instrument for changing society.

Those of us who became social change professionals were not blind to the depth and strength of vested interests in this most vested of nations. We had no illusions about "the enemy." The American political system was recognized as a veil of illusion cast over the brutal reality of corporate interests.

Those of us in government spoke of "guerilla administration," a hit-and-run approach to particular projects involving a floating crap game of change agents in different agencies. There was even an organization known as FEDS, Federal Employees for a Democratic Society, modeled after SDS.

The Metro Center at NIMH, like other branches, had a "study group" of outside consultants whose deliberations and recommendations to the National Advisory Mental Health Council decided which grant applications would be funded. We "broke the rules" of study group appointments by bringing in people of color, individuals with a radical political orientation, and even some nonprofessional activists. There were complaints from some of the more traditional mental health constituencies, but we prevailed and some of our grants had the smack of social change implicit in them. For example, we became involved with the Office of Economic Opportunity in a "manpower development grant" to an organization in Chicago known as the Blackstone Rangers or the Ranger Nation.

The grant was given to a gang. The Rangers were an organization of several hundred black men on the South Side of Chicago who, assisted by a Presbyterian minister named John Fry, could organize up to four thousand demonstrators around the large old church that served as the group's headquarters.

The Rangers were originally one of many basketball and partying groups on turfs in and around the Woodlawn ghetto. They became a different kind of gang when members began to escort "white hunters," men who had come downtown looking for black prostitutes, out of the area. They soon became an informal security force, not unlike the Guardian Angels, but without the sanction of the police and City Hall. When they campaigned on behalf of black activist Dick Gregory's bid for the mayoralty of Chicago and challenged Mayor Daley's South Side machine, the city responded by declaring them a menace. A Gang Intelligence Unit was established by the police department for the purpose of destroying the Rangers by arresting one after another of their leaders on trumped-up charges. Relying on provocateur activity, the police also attempted to start a gang war between the Rangers and the Devil's Disciples, a nearby gang. It was not successful, and a "peace treaty" was signed between the two gangs.

The group's ultimate vindication came after Dr. King's assassination. While the West Side of Chicago suffered a huge and destructive riot, the South Side was calm and controlled. The Rangers patrolled the streets telling people that they should stay cool and not invite police brutality with destructive behavior.

It was this "counter-riot" function of the Rangers that we identified as important and definitive, and in a position paper prepared for the Kerner Commission, we suggested that black and Hispanic youth groups across the country could be seen as a positive and constructive presence in urban ghettos. We found, in similar groups in other cities and in an organization called Y.O.U. (Youth Organizations United), that there was hope for national affiliation, a new base of power in the minority community.

It was not easy to interest political figures and foundations in such a venture. During a meeting we arranged at Urban America, a privately funded think tank on urban affairs, an administrator turned to the head of one of the groups and asked, "What are the purposes of your organization?" The man, a Puerto Rican from New York, began to respond when the door opened and a secretary handed a note to the administrator. Without a word, he abruptly rose and walked out, leaving the rest of us to look at each other for several minutes. When he came back, he sat down and said, "As you were saying . . . ." The gang leader looked directly at him and said, "Hey, man, you ask me a question, then you walk out. What do you call that?"

The administrator suddenly seemed to understand that he had been discourteous. He flushed a bit and said, "Oh, I'm terribly sorry, but that was a call from the chairman of our board, Andrew Heiskell, the head of Time-Life." This was allowed to hang in the air for a moment while the gang leader stared at him and then, in a long, low voice, said, "Shit." No money was forthcoming to Y.O.U. from Urban America.

In *Mau-Mauing the Flak Catchers*, Tom Wolfe used the hip, cynical style American intellectuals love in damning developments with a social conscience. He describes an alleged contact between a black youth group and a white bureaucrat who kowtows to them with a shit-eating grin. In reality, if there had been a bit more respect paid to such spontaneously emerging organizational life—the kind of power sharing that we believed possible in the sixties—the chaotic violence and nihilistic drug use now rampant in the ghettos might have been avoided. For corporate America, the risk was too great.

The war in Vietnam became the central focus of protest and organization by the end of the decade. Some of us attempted to keep the focus on the background issues of race and poverty, the context of a war that was, after all, being fought by the black and the poor against the disempowered poor of another continent. Some of my antiwar colleagues in psychiatry saw themselves as participating in protest activity by writing letters excusing young men from the draft on putative psychiatric grounds. I decided not to do this, as it was in general the more affluent white draft dodgers who were able to obtain such letters, their places in Vietnam to be filled by minorities and poor and working-class whites.

After Nixon's election in 1968 and the subsequent escalation of the war, the energy behind any effort at radical change or even reform of domestic policy was all but dissipated. Nixon's attitude toward community mental health and social psychiatry was predictable. Anything with the words "community" or "social" in it was seen as part of a leftist conspiracy.

Community health is a highly sensitive indicator of political orientation. When Marxist Salvador Allende was elected as president of Chile in 1970, one of his first acts was to establish a network of community health clinics. And when Pinochet and the CIA overthrew him three years later, the clinics were almost immediately dismantled. In a comparable manner, the community mental health movement of the sixties, the legacy of liberalism, was targeted by the Republicans along with other social programs. The original plan of 2,000 comprehensive community mental health centers across the country dissolved in the thin air of reactionary politics, and it was soon evident that sustaining grants for existing mental health centers would be ended and the states would be expected to pick up the tab for ongoing expenses.

The Metro Center learned quite early in the Nixon era that there would be no new money for contracts or grants. During this period, I was involved in antiwar demonstrations and began speaking and writing more directly in opposition to the war. My supervisors were not happy about this, but as long as I added the phrase, "This does not reflect official policy of the National Institute of Mental Health or the Department of Health, Education and Welfare," there was nothing they could do.

I established a personal philosophy of public service around that time, one that has guided my behavior ever since. As long as I was sacrificing opportunities of greater wealth or status by working in government, I would say or write whatever I chose regardless of how offensive that seemed to that government. Bureaucrats are confused and helpless in the face of such an approach. It is not easy to fire someone from a civil service position, and "freedom of speech" is such a sacred phenomenon in this nation that few administrators are prepared to be quoted as saying, "You should not have said that," to a subordinate.

Nevertheless, I was a GS-15-level employee of the federal government, a relatively high rank, and this was the era of COINTELPRO, the FBI program aimed at domestic dissent. At times I became a little paranoid or, at least, that is what my colleagues said when I told them that there were unusual echoes or clicks on the phone when I called home from the office. I learned to think about what paranoia means in the context of legitimate concerns about an illegitimate government. One of my associates simply said that it was the paranoids who were after *him* and left it at that.

To believe that one is being persecuted because of one's importance or centrality in the universe, rather than because of one's group identification or shared attributes, is to be paranoid even if the persecution is real. COINTELPRO attempted to induce paranoia as one of its strategies. It attempted to fragment the Left by creating more distrust than necessary, so that informers would be seen where they did not exist. The FBI also disrupted meetings and attempted to destroy organizations with an insidious form of provocateur activity that pushed any antiestablishment position to an absurd extreme. They were particularly adept at planting ideas that pitted blacks against Jews. It was a program of paranoid reality.

I also became aware of the growing role of social science research in police state functions. It was a revelation of how liberal professionals can minister to fascism. In Pogo's terms, "We have met the enemy and he is us."

Recently the graduating class of a prestigious liberal arts college was presented with a survey questionnaire covered with a letter from the president of the school. The letter encouraged the graduates to answer the questions, which were a follow-up to ones given them on admission four years earlier. It was to be helpful to the university in planning for the future. The letter insisted that the research was in no way an invasion of privacy and, indeed, there was no need for the identity of the student to be revealed.

The principal investigator of this study was a professor of psychology at the University of California at Berkeley named Alexander Astin. Seeing this provided a *deja entendu* experience for me. Twenty years before, Astin was director of research for an organization based in Washington known as the American Council of Education, an organization that sounds innocently pedantic. It is actually the guild of American university and college administrators. Every dean is a member.

Universities are not now known as disinterested institutions dedicated to the pursuit and distribution of "truth." In the sixties, however, the extent to which the university research apparatus was at the service of military and corporate interests was only just becoming evident. We were also slowly becoming aware of the role of the university in creating an ideological hegemony directed at elevating individualism and competitiveness to the pantheon of values and rendering the possibility of collective and redistributive solutions to social problems not only unacceptable but inconceivable. Not until the sixties and only after the student protest movement did most of us discover that the directorship of universities were one and the same as those of corporations. We learned that millions of "endowed" dollars in tax-free ventures represented enormous profits in market manipulations.

This is now a matter of common knowledge even if not a matter of common concern. Then, however, we were shocked that what was thought to be the home of absent-minded professionalism, a kind of lovable, sloppy incompetence, where power, if it existed at all, was vapid, fleeting, pluralistic, and basically well-meaning, was shown to be centralized, relentless, and potentially murderous. The campus protests caused the mask—with its kindly, myopic eyes squinting over threadbare tweed speckled with pipe tobacco—to drop. And we heard the sharp crack of police batons on the heads of children and the National Guard's rifles firing into their very hearts.

At about that time, the American Council of Education decided to "study" campus protest as a social phenomenon, and Alexander Astin designed the research instrument. With the cooperation of the deans of participating colleges, all incoming students were asked to fill out a long and seemingly disjointed questionnaire about their attitudes and experiences. Two years later (this was during the era of almost constant campus activism), the responses on this broad-based interview schedule were correlated with records that revealed actual participation in protest activity, so that a profile of "protest-prone" behavior could be determined with actuarial precision. In other words, based on responses to a nonspecific array of questions, the likelihood of a person's being an activist could be deduced even before they themselves knew it. Most important was the use of group identification patterns rather than individual ones as the basis of prediction. Among Astin's findings was that incoming students with a Jewish name who responded "none" when asked about religious preference were more likely to be troublemakers. If they, in addition, answered "yes" to the question about their ever having tried marijuana, the certainty of future protest behavior was virtually established.

Astin was asked if he were concerned about the possibility that deans of admission might use his research to limit the number of pot-smoking atheistic Jews on campus as a way of preventing protests. He answered that he was just a social scientist and the ultimate use of his research was not his responsibility.

Shrouded with the mantle of value-free science, investigators like Astin were expanding the technologies of social control beyond the wildest imagination of old-fashioned inquisitioners and fascists. They used a kind of mindless research that requires no hypotheses, no imagination, and not much thought, merely large numbers of respondents and computers to do the endless kneading of data. It is the stuff of the Secret Service, which keeps track of seven million potential assassins of the president, and customs officials who check every license plate at every border, and the FBI and CIA sifting through every name and every organization that might offend the status quo. And Astin, now comfortably tenured, is still doing it.

As the sixties came to an end, like the steel door of a vault clanging shut, with a reactionary administration continuing a brutal war begun by a liberal one, with community mental health under a death sentence, and a virtual moratorium on any concern with race relations, poverty, or social and economic justice, I felt it was time to leave Washington.

In the seventies, the culture became preoccupied with shutting down what had been flung open the decade before. Local governments were shocked to find that the community action agencies of the "War on Poverty" thought of themselves as a permanent fixture of urban life. This had to be undone. While traditionally Democratic in nature, city governments happily permitted a Republican administration to eviscerate the federal support structure for OEO programs.

The FBI became obsessed with militant blacks and other domestic revolutionary elements. Either through *agents provocateurs*, harassment at work, direct arrests, or outright murder, it systematically attempted to demoralize, fragment, and destroy the New Left. This was often done under the guise of narcotics control and with the happy cooperation of state and local police authorities.

The hope for an alliance between working-class whites and militant blacks had been destroyed by the assassination of Robert Kennedy and the anti-labor campaigns that pitted whites against blacks. The government encouraged a backlash against affirmative action that continues today in the opposition to "quotas." Antiwar demonstrators were attacked by ostensibly spontaneous demonstrations of men wearing hard hats, who were characterized as working men indignant about the "anti-American" aspects of opposition to the war in Vietnam. Richard Nixon talked about the "forgotten Americans," who were alleged to be working class, patriotic, family-oriented, and religious people fed up with the demands of blacks, hippies, and junkies.

In the meantime, the collectivist and pacifist elements of the sixties were co-opted by ad agencies. "Do it!" a phrase used the decade before to suggest the breaking of cultural shackles, was now used to sell a Caribbean cruise. "Flower Power," once the image of a Buddhist placing a flower in the barrel of an Army gun, became a money-making image for St. Valentine's Day. Bank loans were "revolutionary" and power itself something to find in computers.

By 1970, the momentum of community psychiatry slowed to a halt with the elimination of funds for community mental health centers. Grant funds for socially oriented research became more and more scarce, while money for pharmacological or biologically oriented research became increasingly generous. The texture and complexion of the profession was changing along with the times.

We like to say that we make decisions in life, that we choose to marry or move or become cowboys or priests. We see ourselves steering our little vehicles into something called "the future," a turnpike with an infinity of cloverleaf decision points. A foolish and deceptive culture trains us to think that as individuals we control our destinies and deserve the credit for "achievement" or the blame for "failure." In fact, things happen to us; our paths in life are well laid down by forces of which we have little perception and less understanding. Social class and race are the big ones, invisible hands that open and close the sluices of opportunity with swift, silent movements. Our position in society and the character of the times are the forces that control our lives.

I "decided" to move back to Boston when I was called by the Massachusetts Commissioner of Mental Health and offered a job dealing with drug abuse. It was 1970 and then, as periodically happens when the president needs to distract a nation and blame its victims, there was a "drug epidemic."

The epidemic was not thought to include alcohol and cigarettes, which were as lethal then as they are now. And while the society winked at marijuana and joked about cocaine, which were, in the seventies, upper-class diversions and therefore seemed relatively innocent, it was terrified and outraged about heroin, the sinful drug of the underclass. Nixon declared the "drug menace" to be the "worst threat that ever faced the country."

Massachusetts felt called upon to develop a new set of institutions to deal with the "menace": a treatment and rehabilitation industry to complement and soften the police juggernaut. The governor, Francis Sargent, was a liberal Republican with a reformist administration, much kinder and gentler than anything seen since in Massachusetts and elsewhere in the nation. He sponsored a bill, which soon became law, allowing drug offenders to be directed to treatment facilities instead of going to prison. Such facilities did not yet exist.

Bureaucrats in Massachusetts, as elsewhere, were not hungering for new responsibilities that were not invested with ready cash. A major dispute emerged between the Departments of Mental Health and Public Health about where to locate the new drug rehabilitation authority. The Department of Public Health won, so the new Division of Drug Rehabilitation was created within the Department of Mental Health.

From the outset, much of my work as the "drug commissioner" involved trying to stop other people's plans. In one notable case, a county district attorney tried to tie his political future to the idea of setting up a decommissioned aircraft carrier as a floating drug treatment facility under my command. I was to whistle aboard several thousand junkies and treat them at a comfortable distance from Boston Harbor. The unstated assumption was that if they did not improve, they could be sunk.

I found myself becoming something of a libertarian, never proposing the legalization of drugs as the answer to their abuse, but constantly resorting to a constitutional ideology to ward off some of the impatient suggestions for a psychiatric "final solution." Most of these took the form of recommendations that old TB sanitaria or state hospital wards become the environment for treating this new problem.

But the technologists of social control had fancier ideas to keep track of ever new enemies of the social order. Most of these had to do with information technologies.

The major struggle, and the one that launched my career as a "privacy freak," had to with something called CODAP, which was acronymed into existence by SAODAP, the White House Special Action Office of Drug Abuse Prevention. This was part of the Nixon "War on Drugs." It is interesting the way social problems become transformed into military ones in this society, the "enemy" always being separate, outside, and invasive, as if cancer, poverty, and intoxication were not systemic, built in. The "conquest of space" was the purest expression of this tendency, we the conquerors being, like gods, outside it.

CODAP stood for the Client-Oriented Data Acquisition Process, the "oriented" suggesting once again that the acronym is thought up first, then the title, and finally the program. I described CODAP as a "monster masquerading as a windmill," a cumbersome information system sinuously wrapped around federal drug abuse prevention efforts, with money as the temptation and technological fascism as the eternal, infernal reward.

The teeth of the system was in a "unique identifier," nothing so gross as a tattooed number on the forearm, but allegedly a foolproof method of monitoring and tracking every patient in treatment in the nation. The manifest excuse was that such a system would permit patients on methadone to travel out of state and get their "medicine" from any program in the country without fear of duplication or diversion. Federal law, believe it or not, prohibits the use of the social security number for purposes of identification. The designers of the program considered using fingerprints, but abandoned the idea because of its "connotations." They proposed instead a footprint system of identification, the connotations here being the innocence of the newborn babe. Footprints were reliably and easily obtained from junkies too sedated to know or care that their smelly soles were treading a new path of information technology.

I condensed my concerns about CODAP into a few muted phrases of outraged libertarianism and presented them to the governor's chief administrative assistant, a spiky lawyer and former state representative from Chelsea by the name of Al Kramer. Now a judge in Quincy, Massachusetts, he was then the liberal activist who helped define an ideology and program for his boss. He saw to it that CODAP was described to the governor in the vivid terms of my memo at a time of day when he was most likely to pay attention.

In the meantime, I sent copies of my memo to the drug program directors in the other states. About a half dozen of my counterparts shared my states' rights indignation and went to their bosses as well. A half dozen letters from governors to a federal agency seemed like a ground swell. Governor Sargent, in addition to writing to the president, also penned a note to his cousin, Elliot Richardson, who was secretary of the Department of Health, Education and Welfare. Blood, particularly of a certain refinement, being thicker than the usual sap of politics, had a dramatic effect. Richardson, I was told, called back, saying he was furious that such an outrageous program could have been conceived in an administration of which he was part and that he would see to it that it was stopped.

The footprint identifier was thus stepped on and quietly faded away. Several years later, it was just as quietly replaced by another "unique identifier" of ten numbers deriving from birth date, social security number, and zip code, but by that time the capacity for outrage had been lost.

Soon after I arrived on the job, I was presented with yet another perturbation of bureaucratic peace of mind, a political campaign for the 1970 gubernatorial election. The mayor of Boston, a pseudo-liberal pol named Kevin White, decided to challenge Sargent for the office of governor. As drug abuse was a hot item in the public consciousness, the candidates had to have competing "programs" to deal with the menace. White's advisors opted for methadone maintenance as the treatment of choice and faulted the state for its lack of commitment to an idea that "experts" had defined as the definitive solution to the problem.

Methadone maintenance seemed to me a cynical and racist consignment of an underclass to perpetual dependency, the clinic replacing the pusher with a doctor-cop ambiguity of social control and treatment. As soon as I started talking to addicts, I learned that "patients" on methadone continued to use drugs. Clinic parking lots had become the major copping areas in many towns. "Spit bottles" of unconsumed methadone were selling at $10 a sip. Regardless of the dose of the USP pure narcotic, and regardless of the rituals of urine tests for "illicit" drugs, a majority of the addicts on methadone continued to shoot up with heroin. Almost all of them in addition used whatever analgesics and sedatives were available, including Valium, barbiturates, antihistamines (Phenergan, the favorite), cough medicine (Tussionex, the winner here), paregoric, Percodan, and, of course, booze.

While the liberal and libertarian types liked methadone maintenance as a means of controlling drug abuse while taking an incremental step toward legalization, both the fundamentalist Right and the revolutionary Left opposed it. This represented a political realignment, a new populism of sorts, involving a Left-Right coalition against centrist, professionalized, entrenched, and basically conservative elitism.

When I was called into the governor's office and asked what his program should be, I offered an alternative that was more ideologically pure and (to me) politically palatable: self-help.

Self-help was a vestige of the sixties, community-based, egalitarian, nonbureaucratic, and youthful. It was voluntaristic and cheap, to appeal to the Republicans. There were a few prototypical programs in the state, ranging from hip, scraggly drop-in centers to long-term residential treatment programs modeled on Synanon and Daytop Village. The latter, closing a small circle for me in my community psychiatry sojourn, were called "therapeutic communities," though their leaders knew little if anything about Maxwell Jones and did not much care for or about psychiatrists in any case. The natural leadership skills of many of the formerly addicted were permitted to flourish in these programs, and, while suspicious of professionals and bureaucrats, they soon saw the governor and me as allies.

The governor's first TV campaign spot showed him (uncharacteristically) in his shirtsleeves, saying to the camera, "If you were a 15-year-old with a drug problem, would you want to talk to a 50-year-old bureaucrat? I'm going to make it possible for young people to help other young people with drug problems so they can work together to rid their communities of the menace of drugs." His advisors had calculated that Sargent's Yankee, patrician stiffness was a handicap in a race against a younger and more ethnic urbanite.

I was not actually asked to campaign for him, which would have been against the law for a civil servant, but various "public education" conferences organized by the governor's office were attended by audiences bearing Sargent buttons. I think I may have been the entertainment for several fund-raising dinners.

Sargent's appointees had a social change orientation. His Commissioner of Youth Services promised to unshackle the children in youth detention centers. His Commissioner of Welfare had alliances with welfare rights organizations. His Commissioner of Public Health had been a publisher of an alternative newspaper, and his Commissioner of Corrections believed in furloughs, prisoners' rights, and community-based correctional programs. Later, a reorganization created a Secretary of Human Services, and reform was slowed down by the pure weight of bureaucracy.

No sooner was a $4 million drug bill enacted than another sacred tradition of Massachusetts politics slipped out from under the rocks. A legislator called to congratulate me on the appropriation, for which, he added, he had voted. Then he said, "There's a fine old doctor in my community who is retiring from a career of general practice. I would appreciate it if you would arrange a contract with him to develop a drug abuse prevention program."

Some of my advisors had told me that this is the way things were done, a simple system of favors and credits. But I came with a protective mechanism borrowed from NIMH, a "study group" of outside consultants to advise on the distribution of grants and contracts. I assembled a "Drug Program Review Board," comprised largely of self-help advocates, but also including professionals such as doctors and lawyers, whose purpose was to review applications from community groups and make recommendations on how to fund them. Board members were appointed by the governor. When legislators called, I would thank them for their interest and say that I would be sure to share their concern with the Board. The usual response was an uncomfortable silence, after which I would hear something like "What the fuck is *that*?"

Things otherwise did not go smoothly. As I was about to sign the contracts for the hundred or so original self-help programs we helped to organize, I was informed by one of the business managers in the Department of Mental Health that he could not "sign off" on these contracts because, in his opinion, they were unconstitutional. Neither I nor the commissioner could prevail over his conclusion that organizations which had peace signs on their walls were politically active, and ones run by renegade priests in the basements of churches were religious organizations, and that contracts with political or religious groups were a violation of the Commonwealth's highest law.

Now it can be told. The problem of his overscrupulousness was solved with a bottle of 12-year-old Scotch. That and similar experiences led me to the formulation of a now universally ignored principle of public administration, which the reader is free to call *Dumont's Law of Expanding Negativity*. According to its precepts, people working in bureaucracies are not aware of their existence except by exerting a negative influence. They are not acknowledged or appreciated for facilitating their piece of a complex process, such as signing off on a contract. If they act expeditiously, they remain invisible and unknown. If, however, they procrastinate or construct an impediment to the process, if they say "No!" someone, somewhere, is likely to acknowledge that they exist. The larger the organization, the more necessary is the need for acknowledgment, and the more obstructive is the effect of any single negative influence. The larger the bureaucracy, the more the negativity, and the more destructive each negative act is—a whole ecology of people trying to affirm themselves through mutual denial.

In any case, I personally do not know of another instance in the annals of public administration in which an entire substance abuse program was facilitated by a bottle of whiskey.

Another troublesome issue at the outset had to do with sex. A dropout from Daytop Village rented a storefront in Boston, installed a few cots, and established a "program." He was able to recruit a number of addicts and actually assisted them to a drug-free state with a half-baked therapeutic community. When his program's application for a contract came before the Review Board, one of the Board members, who was active in the "T.C." movement, said that he had heard rumors that the director was exacting sexual favors from female residents.

The director was invited in for a discussion which was unlike most study group deliberations.

"Jimmy D'Amato told me that you're fucking residents in your program."

"Jimmy D'Amato is a fucking liar."

"You're full of shit. They used to call you 'the kissing junkie' at Daytop before you split. And you split because you couldn't keep your hands off your cock."

"Yeah, well, at Walpole [Prison], you couldn't keep your fuckin' hands off anybody else's cock."

And so forth.

Having satisfied ourselves after this discussion and a site visit that the program did not meet even *our* flexible standards for self-help, we then had the problem of what to do with it. Even its most vociferous opponents on the Board agreed that there were a dozen or so drug-free addicts in the place, who were not only fiercely loyal but would probably end up back on the streets if the program were closed down. In the end, the decision was to give them a small "survival" grant with the suggestion that the director leave for another state.

It made no sense, but it worked out much later. First, the director in question organized his clients to picket my office and give interviews on talk shows about how Dumont and Sargent were not really supportive of self-help. I could deal with my own ruffled ego feathers, but not the governor's before an election. Kramer, the governor's assistant, called and wanted to know what the furor was all about. He said that to avoid further embarrassment to the governor's program, I should explain the true facts to the public.

This was our first and only real argument. I had been running around the state, appearing on television and at public meetings, trying to establish the respectability of self-help, baptizing ex-addicts and school dropouts with the leased authority of psychiatry and state bureaucracy. If it emerged that sex was going on in one of these programs, the public's worst fantasies would be realized. This was long before the revelations of how many of the most respectable psychiatrists in the most respectable mental hospitals were screwing their patients. I decided that the best thing to say was nothing and simply responded, "No comment," when journalists called to ask about the project in question. Journalists soon get bored and the public forgets. Before long, the existence of a state program of substance abuse control supporting community self-help programs staffed by nonprofessionals was a matter of routine.

But a methadone constituency was rapidly developing in the state, and it was not long before the struggle between self-help and methadone became the major issue. The former was hip, radical, and black, the latter academic, pragmatic, and professionalized. It was also city versus state—as the Boston program was oriented entirely around methadone.

At one time during our struggle, there were four different sets of auditors going through our books looking for trouble. This included a congressional audit initiated, we opined, through some of Boston's contacts with Speaker of the House Tip O'Neill's office. It felt like harassment, but nothing embarrassing was to be found. The Boston tradition was that a program director resigned just before the auditors arrived. I had tacitly decided some time earlier that if I were going to be a guerilla administrator, to use my profession as an instrument of social change, I would not let myself be vulnerable to charges of being self-serving. Perhaps revolutionaries, like physicians, have a higher responsibility to be moral than others not because they are more moral people but because there is more at stake.

The acme of our efforts was the development of MASH, the Massachusetts Association of Self-Help, which we organized and financed. In 1973, MASH sponsored a three-day conference at Brandeis University characterized by a heady mixture of radical politics and chaos. There was a black caucus and an Hispanic caucus and a therapeutic community caucus and a "legalize pot" caucus. A fistfight erupted when a T.C.er said that he could be sent back to prison for being in the same room with a pot smoker, and the smoker shouted that we had to "smash the system." There was even a rumor of a gun in someone's possession.

Governor Sargent was coming to the meeting, and a statement had to be drafted to present to him. Listening to the endless discussions, I managed to condense all the passion and ideology of the three days into the classic single page of prose beyond which chief executives lose interest. Minutes before the governor arrived, the statement was read out loud and throatily approved by the attendees. When he walked in, everybody in the room came to their feet and started cheering. He was a little startled by the enthusiasm and could not have guessed that it was more for themselves than for him. The ovation lasted about ten minutes.

Following a few perfunctory remarks of greeting and good wishes, the governor listened politely while the statement was read to him by a former addict. It was a nice moment—a governor listening to a junkie talking about the defects in a social system that cause personal pathology and the need for a redistribution of power and the creation of increasingly large and comprehensive systems of mutual support. The governor seemed intrigued with the thoughtfulness of the statement, if not for its call for a social revolution, and said he intended to study it more carefully. He turned to me to thank me for my role, but as he did, he did another double take from the sudden volume of cheers that broke out across the room.

Almost on cue, another politician strode in. John Buckley was sheriff of Middlesex County and had been featured on the cover of *Time* magazine as a law officer who wanted to outlaw guns. He was considering a challenge to Sargent as head of the state's Republican party and for the governorship. He sat down with a broad smile after waving to the crowd, and Sargent went back to the podium to say, "I want to welcome Sheriff Buckley and assure him that the cheers were not for him but for Dr. Dumont."

Sargent was replaced in 1972 by Michael Dukakis in the anti-Republican backlash of Watergate. The bright possibilities of self-help were soon dragged down under the weight of professionalism and government cost cutting. The budget for self-help programs was cut to the bone along with other social programs, and, before long, the methadone constituency triumphed. It was time for me to leave both drug rehabilitation and administration. I began looking for a community clinic in which to practice what I had been trained in and was prepared to do all along, community psychiatry.

In 1975, I found it.

FOUR

There is a texture to a city. Sights, sounds, smells, the undulations of sidewalk and street, the stop and go of movement become confluent in a pattern that is almost tactile. Paris feels more silky, more sinuous than New York, where the sough of a million manhole covers and claxons, the hard-edge slashes of steel and glass in a dwindling sky, and the dogs of war unleashed at every traffic crossing give the city even in its most meandering moments the feel of sandpaper.

Not that an abrasive touch is always unwelcome. After driving for hours through rolling hills covered with varying shades of green, one's eyes are drawn magnetically, maybe hungrily, to a car dump. Everything is a matter of context and scale.

Chelsea, Massachusetts, is small and rough, a shard. On Broadway, one is met by a loose weave of aggressive drivers proud of the illusion of unrestricted personal mobility, though often quite bound to Chelsea. Woofers are mounted behind grills that blast the sounds of salsa or Southeast Asian rock. Tires screech as drivers drag race from one diffident stoplight to another.

A vicious territoriality surrounds these cars. Parking spaces are claimed with trash cans, as if assigned to the residents of triple deckers. The city seems always on the verge of a riot; a fight over a parking space is a likely precipitant.

A *West Side Story-Romeo and Juliet* sexuality pervades the atmosphere, highlighted by flashes of blade and bullet. Girls—children, really—of a different ethnicity are always fair game for male adolescent lust and the fury of the offended mother tongue.

The nights cry havoc in Chelsea: shouts, knifings, rape, and fire. Small as it is, Chelsea is the "Fire Capital of America." Its history is written in fire. In the nineteenth century, Chelsea was a spa for proper Bostonians. Residents of the Back Bay and Beacon Hill ferried over to bathe in the

Chelsea Creek, now nearly gelid and stinking with chemicals.

A century ago, Chelsea was pristine. Today, the wrecks of handsome homes, their widows' walks long abandoned, overlook the oil tanks, waste disposal plants, and junkyards that line the city's coast.

Chelsea has also become the "Junk Capital of America." How could this gracious, seaside village, the stuff of Currier and Ives prints (a white-steepled church and the cozy homes of its parishioners circled by a pair of rolling hills), become a gigantic junkyard?

It was the wrack of progress, coastal urban tides washing up to higher ground. At the end of the nineteenth century, there was a major fire in Boston, attributed to Jewish junk dealers in an irresistible mixture of anti-Semitism and reality. There was at that time a transiently reformist, "good government" city administration in power, i.e., a Yankee, anti-immigrant one, which wasted no time in enacting what was perceived as the most progressive urban legislation in America, the first zoning ordinance. Junkyards, and only incidentally their Jewish owners, were banned from Boston. In one abrupt move, several hundred Jewish families relocated their homes and businesses to sleepy Chelsea. Overnight, it became a Jewish city, the Junk Capital of America, and soon the Fire Capital of America.

Fire fighters all over the world know about the periodic conflagrations in Chelsea, from the 1908 fire to the one in 1973, when 18 square blocks went up in flames.

Fire is still a terrifying presence in Chelsea, one of the most densely populated cities in the country. It is congested with ancient multiple-family dwellings, each unit of which is often occupied by multiple families.

Chelsea, like most poor communities, is a city of smokers. It is also a major drug connecting locus for the Northeast, and like everywhere else, alcoholism is rampant.

And there is arson. Not the affair of crazed, enuretic fire fiends masturbating at the sight of a house in flames, it is the business of business—money. Insurance scams play a minor role, as most of the community is considered uninsurable. Arson in Chelsea has more to do with the phenomenon of gentrification, which has systematically taken shelter from the poor in one city after another and given it, when it is given at all, to the middle class.

Until quite recently, Chelsea was spared from the real estate parasites. They were busy in Charlestown and the South End and Beacon Hill, transforming rooming houses and tenements into the urban dream homes of the upwardly mobile. The heady incline in real estate prices promised instant wealth. A house became transformed from a place to live into a commodity to buy and sell. And since the higher the rate of inflation, the higher the profit, banks, insurance companies, and even medical centers and universities found that investment in housing provided the quickest and largest return on their dollars.

Emptied of its former tenants, with some new plaster and paint and aluminum windows thrown on, what was once the home of low-income tenants became a half-million-dollar condo. Speculators did not worry about whether or not the condos actually sold, because with tax write-offs, short-term depreciation, and as equity for yet more loans, the buildings were more profitable as empty high-priced condos than occupied low-income apartments.

The market was driven by a "grow or die" mentality. Like a car with a fouled carburetor, unless it kept accelerating, it would stall. Areas of old houses provided the fuel for this internal combustion system in the process of burning itself out. And despite Chelsea's reputation for junk and junkies and for fires, the gentrifiers were forced eventually to come across the Mystic-Tobin Bridge connecting Boston to Chelsea.

As recently as a decade ago, a house could be bought in the city for $20,000. Apartments, lavish in size, though rundown and poorly maintained, were cheap and available. With Section 8 and Chapter 707, the federal and state subsidized housing programs, even welfare recipients could rent a comfortable apartment.

Then, during the eighties, like a blitzkrieg, block after block was bought up by unknown corporate buyers. Family after family was evicted, or their rents were suddenly jacked up. This is where homelessness comes from. It does not come out of the blue; it is the result of real estate transactions designed by and for the greedy.

Tenants do not like to give up their homes, and housing law in Massachusetts is not entirely on the side of the landlord. A competent lawyer, such as those working for Greater Boston Legal Services, a residue of the War on Poverty, can prevent an eviction for at least six months.

This is where the arsonist comes in, often an unemployed teenager or junkie promised big bucks for setting a small fire. No one really wants anyone to die, but after a bit of smoke damage, a suddenly vigorous housing inspector determines that a house is no longer habitable and must be vacated immediately. Gentrification proceeds.

If the house is insured, so much the better, but insurance adjustors can be a nuisance with "fires of suspicious origin," and, in any case, the big money is in buying and borrowing based on inflated values.

Fire, unfortunately, has a way of getting out of hand. Even a small one, designed for just the right amount of smoke damage, can sometimes kill. Every mother in Chelsea goes to bed with the ever-present fear that her children will burn to death during the night.

But there is a slower death attendant upon the fires of Chelsea. It has to do with the element of lead, the base metal on which the new Chelsea was built. Much of junk is lead. It is eminently meltable and malleable and hence recyclable into its many uses: bullets, toy soldiers, pipes for gas (if no longer for water), and as ground for the pigment in paint. Lead is a "good" ground for pigments because it is cheap, opaque, and permits an intense saturation of color. It also expands and contracts smoothly with temperature changes and so tends not to crack, making it ideal for external surfaces.

Ship paint is about 90 percent lead. The shipyards on the harbor were traditionally the unofficial source of much low-cost, do-it-yourself decoration and several generations of poisoned children.

Lead does not break down. It goes nowhere chemically. When old houses with a half century or so of repeated coatings of lead paint go up in flames, the ashes sink into the soil and dust of the city to last . . . forever.

When the streets of America became home to the automobile, lead batteries came to Chelsea's junkyards to end their days. These too would feed the flames of the city's fires, so that more and more lead would be silted up in the dust of the city.

Lead kills insidiously most of the time. Even the high blood pressure that comes much later as the result of kidney damage is silent and often enough heralded only by a stroke in one's final hours. Like a sadistic murderer, lead does not kill nerve cells quickly and outright, but maims them, so that a limp wrist or a colicky bowel or a misunderstood homework assignment are more often its symptoms than acute brain damage and death.

But death occurs. The daily consumption of a chip of lead paint the size of a child's fingernail for a mere month can kill. The occasional lollipop dropped in a playground and put back into the child's mouth can destroy his or her blood and brain, the latter forever.

The treatment is hardly a treatment. "Chelating agents" are chemicals that bind with lead in the blood, permitting its excretion through the kidneys. But they themselves can be toxic to the kidneys. Also, since with chronic exposure the lead has been deposited in the bones and remains in equilibrium with the blood, chelation often results in a sudden rise in the blood lead level as it is mobilized from the bones. Not infrequently, it is after such "treatment" that a sudden burst of lead in the blood reaches a high enough level to cause brain damage that had not existed before.

There is no normal level of lead in the body. Any amount is too much, as there is a straight-line relationship between the amount of lead at even very low levels and measurable degrees of disturbed behavior or learning difficulties. So the fires of Chelsea go on killing and injuring people long after they are put out. But the memory of a great fire is often extinguished with its flames, because the population is ever changing.

Chelsea is no longer a Jewish city. A generation after Operation Bootstrap, Chelsea became the port of entry for a whole new population of migrants from Puerto Rico. They came from the Western rim, from villages and farms that were ignored by the neocolonial industrial development in the capital.

They came to the densest city in America, Yankee-Jewish, industrial, and racist. The culture shock of urban America hit hard and fast. A teenage girl who came home from school wearing lipstick was called a *puta*, a whore, a label that could only be removed by an early marriage.

The schools, like cultural pseudomorphs, rigid and incapable of change, could not accept the reality that upwardly mobile, impoverished Jews were no longer using them as the jumping board to the middle class. They remained "academic" and monolingual and all but invited their Puerto Rican students to drop out by the tenth grade.

If pregnancy represented the opportunity to drop out of school for the girls, dealing drugs did the same for the boys. Marijuana, heroin, pills of varying sedative-hypnotic-analgesic composition packaged as "pacs," TCP, and cocaine—including its devastatingly efficient "cracked" variety—were added to the rivers of alcohol and Tester's Glue, creating a fictive solution to the emptiness and futurelessness of foreclosed lives. Much more money could be made as a low-order dealer, a "mule" carrying drugs, than in the stifling factories where men and women worked long hours in blind-alley jobs.

As early as 1970, when I became the drug commissioner, Chelsea was already known as one of the major "drug-copping" spots in the Boston metropolitan area. It has since been described as the major port-of-call for illegal drugs for the entire Northeast. Chelsea has always been a city of superlatives.

During the seventies, it became the poorest city in the state, as well as the densest, the most lead-poisoned, and the most unemployed. "Chelsea Pride," the bumper stickers read, something of a joke because the very name Chelsea (like Hoboken or Brooklyn when announced as the provenance of a guest on an old radio show) would bring a little laugh of contempt from other North Shore residents. There was little pride in Chelsea. Its leadership was fleeting, and as often as not, fleeing from auditors. Whenever there was big money to be spent or made on "development," for example, the housing on Admiral's Hill, once the site of a U.S. naval hospital, or the shopping malls that sprouted like weeds, there was a tradition of the "gentlemanly thing to do." Gentlemen gave big tips, and not a few palatial homes were built far from Chelsea on the kickbacks arranged there.

Occasionally the city would be the subject of national media attention. It seemed to have to go up in flames in order to be treated seriously. Otherwise, when mentioned on national news, it was as if for comic relief.

On one occasion, the chair of the school committee brought Chelsea its 15 minutes of fame by demanding that the high school librarian remove and presumably burn a book containing the word *fuck*. A poem had been assigned to a literature class that described the quality of urban Puerto Rican adolescent life, and the offensive expletive was used *en passant*. A parent complained, and Chelsea was soon held up to the nation, as if by the tail or by the ear, with that curl of contempt which characterizes the offended libertarianism of a free press. (Is it not true, by the way, that in more than a century of its august history, the *New York Times* has not once permitted that word to appear between its sheets?)

The school committee chair was indeed a bully. Once a mayor who fretted and strutted his hour on the stage of Chelsea politics, he continued to dominate its educational system and was the hard-hitting editor-owner-publisher-chief reporter for its paper of record, the *Chelsea Record.* He was, in a sense, the chatelaine of the town's literacy and used the paper's front page as a personal "I've been thinking . . ." column. He believed it was his personal responsibility to savor or dismiss words in print unsuited to the delicate palates of Chelsea's youth. Perhaps he believed that if he, like the *New York Times*, could keep the word *fuck* out of print, the children of the city would not use the word or even do the deed.

The underside of Chelsea came into the fleeting, fitful light of national media attention a few years later, following what came to be called "the King Arthur fracas." This perturbation of Camelot took place in the Chelsea Produce Center, the largest in New England. Kiwis from California, mangoes from Haiti, grapes from Chile, apples from New Zealand, hot-house tomatoes, manioc, and Maine potatoes—almost anything that can be grown anywhere on earth and trucked, shipped, or flown anywhere else—come to the warren of sheds and truck depots of the Chelsea Produce Center.

It was a part of the city that never slept, and at 4 a.m. every day, gears ground, crates crashed, and polyphonic, polyglotic shouts and curses were exchanged in the riot of frenzied activity that underlay the quotidian calm of salads to come.

Frenzy demands its due. There was a motel on the grounds of the Produce Center. It was not a place for children, nor was it a franchise of any of those national firms that have come to call a plastic-lined, cinder-block room a "holiday" place or a thing of "quality" or the very "best" the Western world has to offer. The King Arthur Motel, its pretensions to ancient English royalty notwithstanding, was a place for the desperate rest and recreation of the tough men who tendered fruit. It was a place for heavy drinking and lightly clad or non-clad women; the vestigial traces of New England puritanism, the pasties and the G-string, were dropped at the King Arthur. Nude dancing was truly nude dancing, and predictably the rooms were available for the denouement after the high-decibel, spot-lit bump-and-grind foreplay in the lounge.

Predictable also was the presence of an element to whom the press relegates the word "organized" as if it belonged nowhere else: criminals, racketeers, gangsters—the Mob. The Chelsea police respected the place. But the police from the adjacent town of Everett, a few blocks away, were another matter. One of their number dropped in on a casual, off-duty mission of lust.

One of the gangsters at the bar was thought to be connected to the death of a relative or friend of the police officer. Words were exchanged, conceivably including the one barred by the chair of the school committee. The cop called his friends and, before long, Camelot found itself under siege by the Everett Police Department. Moat and drawbridge, poignard and petard were helpless before the invading army, which crashed through the gate, trampling over the groaning board, spilling bottles of sack as boars' heads dropped to the floor, halberds clattered, and maidens fled behind the arras.

The Chelsea police eventually arrived, as such events are often picked up on their scanners. But confused by the ideological ambiguities of the struggle and having, let's face it, split loyalties, they did little more than stand by to maintain order while the Everett police systematically trashed the place, beat every civilian they could lay their batons on, and finally crashed through one bedroom after another until they found the prime suspect cowering under a bed on which was a naked lady doing her nails. He was dragged out and killed, or maybe he died from a heart attack; the legalistic details are obscure.

The whole thing was considered a failure of police protocol. Some officers were actually sent to prison. The innocent bystanders on the Chelsea force were suspended for a while, as they should have done "something," according to the argument. And for several days, Chelsea was in the news again.

On yet another occasion, the city gained some media attention beyond its borders when its mayor decided that if the governor could be attended by a state police officer, then he, as mayor, deserved to be driven and protected by one of Chelsea's police officers. The chief of police, a pragmatic man whose thin blue line of subordinates was already overwhelmed by the demands of routine mayhem, declined to provide the mayor his escort, so the mayor fired him. The chief refused to leave his office, which led to a complicated battle of administrative law, which was never quite resolved.

Chelsea's mayor serves a two-year term, an arrangement that allows for bare minutes of urban governance between bouts of electioneering.

This particular mayor was not the only volatile personality to bring

Chelsea into the national news. John Silber, the president of Boston University, decided to claim Chelsea's feeble, overwhelmed, and inadequate, but quite public school system as property of his university. He had previously bid to take over the City of Boston's school system, but underestimated the determination of the politicians, parents, and teachers of a major city to manage their children's education.

For Silber, it was a matter of ideology as well as providing his school and himself some play in the press. He believed in the efficiency of privately managed enterprises and that the "intelligence" residing in the university could solve any social problem. His personal style of management had resulted in one of the most bitter faculty strikes ever seen on a campus, but he believed that a tough regimen could snap Chelsea's drugged and pregnant dropouts into proper, productive, law-abiding citizens like his students at Boston University.

Silber's campaign of academic imperialism finally triumphed over the objections of the unions and spokespeople for the minority population of Chelsea. After losing a temperamental bid for the governorship of Massachusetts, he planted B.U.'s flag in the heart of what was left of Chelsea Pride.

It was a protracted death agony. Later, with the city's funds exhausted, and teachers, fire fighters, police officers, and garbage collectors seeing payless paydays, the mayor of Chelsea approached the mayor of Boston to discuss the possibility of a merger. Boston graciously declined.

When the city was finally declared bankrupt in the fall of 1991, instead of bailing Chelsea out with state revenues, Governor William Weld (who had defeated Silber) appointed a receiver. The city once again was the subject of national media attention, humiliated, having lost any semblance of control over its own affairs.

I started work in Chelsea in the fall of 1975. I remembered standing on a suburban hill two years earlier and a dozen miles away during the last "great" fire in Chelsea, while a column of smoke rose straight up from what seemed a bombed city.

To get to the Chelsea Community Counseling Center, one crossed the bridge and took the third Chelsea exit, marked "Webster Avenue." The first exit was almost mid-span and meandered dizzily down from the bridge to the Produce Center. The second, where the bridge hit ground level, was marked "Business District." But just before Route 1 lost itself in the wilds of Revere, there was one last chance to reach Chelsea.

Webster Avenue skirted a shopping plaza with a Bradlees department store, a Walgreens drugstore, a liquor store, a few fast-food eateries, and—a surprise—a movie theater.

Now closed, the Parkway Plaza Cinema then had two screens devoted to the "XXX" variety of pornography: all kisses, no hugs. I was later to join forces with the Salvation Army in an effort to remove this center of culture. Captain Lloyd thought the space would make a lovely community recreation room. I thought that a different brand of movie might be shown, possibly about race relations, collective resistance to oppression, or the future of the Third World—films uplifting in a less concrete sense than "Sex-Starved Stewardesses." Neither of our fantasies was to be realized. Home videos succeeded in ridding Chelsea of its only movie theater; the building now remains empty and shut tight against any recreational purpose.

Nestled between the back of Bradlees and Route 1 was one of the town's public housing projects, its impoverished residents endlessly teased by the backside of a mall and the promises of the open road. To drive, to buy, perchance to dream, was the lot of residents of the Locke Street project.

The project and two others, Clinton Court and Guam Road, were built on or near the Chelsea Creek. They were constructed of brick and cinder block, resulting in a "wick effect" by which moisture is sucked from the creek below. Moss grew on the walls and along the bronchial mucosa of the asthmatic children who lived there.

High on a hill, across Webster Avenue from the Parkway Plaza Mall, was the Chelsea Soldiers' Home, one of two in the state built when public money was available, health and domiciliary care were still bargains, and veterans were okay in everybody's book. The Chelsea Soldiers' Home perched San Simeon-like on the highest hill in the city. Three wings stretched toward Boston from the main building, and when the setting sun glittered golden in its windows, it seemed like a Hindu goddess in hard times. If one were a veteran and "knew somebody," one could get free medical care and shelter for life. It was an open secret that many of the vets domiciled at the Soldiers' Home would routinely saunter down the hill to the bars of the city's demi-monde.

In the bars, as everywhere else in Chelsea, the TV sets are on all the time. TV's earnest, endless selling, its matter-of-fact reiteration of events that have no existence outside of its own reality, its velleities masquerading as lust, its stop-action verisimilitude of life and time, is everywhere.

I visited the home of a family in which a 21-year-old woman had hung herself the day before. Grief, rage, longing, guilt were suffused with the blaring sounds of a hysterical daytime quiz show. The laughter and applause from a happy audience hung in the air like satanic mockery. Family members were reluctant to turn the set off during our talk.

The children of Chelsea walk and talk like cartoon animals. Their mothers are as absorbed with the vicissitudes of soap-opera lives as with their own. And the elderly? I went to see a patient in a nursing home. As I was leaving, I passed a room off the lobby called "The Rec Room." (What snide, sadistic humor had gone into the printing of that sign?) Eight or ten residents were tied to chairs around the perimeter of the room. Against one wall was a huge TV screen, playing at a very high volume. Not one of the posey-belted old men and women was watching the screen, but they seemed to be nodding, possibly even vibrating, in preconscious synchronicity to the flicker of sight and sound in the room. It was a *perfusion* of television, another view, I thought, of hell.

Beyond the bars, however, a block after Broadway at the corner of Webster and Spencer Avenues, was the simple white church whose basement would become the center of my professional life.

Even if one were tempted to use the main entrance, behind a wrought iron gate, up a few Baptist-modest steps to the tightly shut doors of the Horace Memorial Church, one would have been stopped by the hieratic notice board on the wall. Under the name of the church and a list of the hours of services were the stark words, "MENTAL HEALTH IS AROUND THE CORNER."

I was charmed by the statement and I remain warmed by its memory. The minister was a man of pedestrian imagination, and I do not believe he would have chuckled to himself like a Barry Fitzgerald-type village priest at the ambiguity of the phrase. I suspect that he meant that visitors to the Chelsea mental health clinic should not stress the hinges and timbers of the locked doors to the sanctuary with psychotic perseverance. He was a Sunday morning moonlighter, showing up at other times of the week in a

Hawaiian shirt to complain about the mess in the bathroom shared by the church and clinic. He acted more like a landlord than a steward of the House of the Lord, with little sense of a Christian mission to the mentally ill in having the clinic in the basement.

I was greeted by a committee of the staff in the kitchen, which I soon learned served as the conference room, staff lounge, day treatment center, and occupational therapy room. They were not particularly cordial and finally asked the question that underlay their reserve. "How long do you intend to stay? Can we count on you for at least a year?"

They surmised that I was merely idling between high-powered jobs, or worse, collecting information for a quick book. They found it difficult to believe that I was prepared to spend a significant portion of my brilliant career in this kitchen. But I was to stay for 16 years, remaining there after all of the original cast of characters, including the landlordly minister, had left. I was eventually forced to leave, laid off as a state employee when the clinic was swept up in the dark cloud of "privatization," the sacrament of the last living god, the Market. But I'm running ahead of my story.

I did not have an office. No one had an office. There were four rooms thinly divided by plasterboard, which the various disciplines—psychiatry, social work, nursing, and psychology—had claimed as territories like jungle animals with their droppings. A stethoscope and blood pressure machine were in the doctors' room, an old MMPI form in the psychologists' space, and so forth.

At times when the clinic was busy, staff would scurry about looking for a place in which to interview a patient. There were a couple of chilly rooms upstairs, the Sanctuary itself (a little daunting for guilt-ridden patients) and rarely, because frowned upon by the other staff, the kitchen.

There was a yard outside with a few balding patches of grass gone to seed. During the summer, clinicians could be seen talking to patients there. This would not satisfy the most rigorous standards of confidentiality, as passersby on Spencer Avenue could witness an interaction different from normal conversation; i.e., someone was really listening to someone else.

The Christianity of the place was rarely a problem. We once requested that the Sunday school teachers not leave the walls plastered with life-sized pictures of Jesus. After some grumbling, they eventually complied.

A functional community mental health center staff complains about the lack of space without much conviction. The clinic itself is only the axis around which revolves a centrifugal pattern of activity. Patients are seen at home for the slightest of reasons, and a network of consultation with other agencies of "caretakers" in town exists, so that much if not most of the work is done outside clinic walls.

Home visits are not just for the aged, paralyzed, dying, or neurotically housebound. A patient will speak differently at home. There, he or she is in his or her proper domain and you are the subject matter, the guest, perhaps an honored or intimidating one, possibly even a fearful one, but a guest nonetheless. One's house, one's "things," and the other lives, human or otherwise, that permeate them are as much a part of a person as the secrets he or she chooses to share. Trying to perform a psychiatric examination in a hospital or a clinic is like trying to listen to a symphony by talking to the musicians. They may be insightful and descriptive, but they are only words, fragments of something larger and more complex. The way a pet is treated, the fact that the television is always on, the way people shout to one another or remain silent, the mess or the neatness, the objects celebrated or disdained, the noise in the halls, and a thousand other details are more revealing about the reality of a person's emotional life than a dream of exquisite clarity and poignancy. Mind is not an object or a container but a network of relationships.

I had an early revelation about my own site-specific behavior as a community psychiatrist in Chelsea. (In the clinic, I was "the doctor"; whatever I said was guided by a sense of responsibility.) I left the clinic one afternoon shortly after I came to Chelsea. As I was walking down the street to my car, I passed a group of boys about the uncharming age of 12 or so sitting on a stoop. The 12-year-old Chelsea male is a formidable and implacable enemy of civilization. Encased in grunts and laughter was a half-greeting to the square grown-up in tie and jacket marching by, something like, "Whereyagoin' foureyes?"

I was thrust into a time warp. Einstein's clock chimed and rattled at infinite speed, clattering and shattering onto Brooklyn schoolyard cement almost a half century earlier. Within the space of the same moment (surely, at that speed, space and time are the same), my preadolescent arm flew upward and the first, second, fourth, and fifth digits of the left hand began to contract.

The camera stopped. The voice-over, sounding perhaps too much like Charlton Heston, spoke with deliberate, studied casualness.

"You are not yourself 12 years of age. They are sitting there with frozen sneers waiting for you to reveal to the frightened, bewildered faces just below the surface what they think is true but hope is not: that all adults are children like them. They are not your patients, but they could be and may yet be. You have the opportunity to show them that with all our lies and defects, grown-ups are more adult than children and it is a good and noble thing to become one."

Charlton Heston as Moses or God or one's own presumptuous ego can be convincing if not irresistible. Before the camera could begin again, the hand of the raised arm gave a friendly, open half-flight of a wave, an over-the-shoulder greeting from an easier, less-threatened, less-threatening world than these poor kids knew. (Maybe someday they will remember.)

It was a small epiphany, not unlike that of Jean Valjean when he stepped on a child's 40-*sou* piece with the instinct of a thief and saw the instinct wither and disappear into thin air at the memory of a gift. I realized that being a community psychiatrist was a little like being a priest or a rabbi. One wore one's role all the time, and its purposes could be as truly realized in an offhand moment, a fleeting gesture, a smile of tolerance, the smallest of cares, as it could be during hours of ritualized professionalism.

The ego is that part of Dr. Freud's tripartite brain which is the steward of civilization, an observing, patient, integrating, Taoist leader, which neither commands nor seduces. It may be homesick for that ancient golden age of hunter-gatherers when life was a shared business, but for now the ego is the only adult show in town. Psychiatrists model ego behavior, or should. In therapy, we should create an environment slightly more muted than the rest of the world, one less hysterical and less menacing. Psychiatrists and other therapists should not be too fancy, too clever or cute, and while their offices can have a personality, the environment should make the patient feel that he or she has entered nothing so grand as Radio City Music Hall or a New Orleans bordello.

The psychotherapist asks questions out of genuine curiosity, and if that curiosity is legitimate and compelling, the patient can come to share it. The patient cannot ask questions about him- or herself without immediately moving into a more emotionally mature position. Such questions are asked from slightly beyond the hot seat of longing and guilt. They are asked tolerantly, without the self-hatred with which we all seem to have been endowed.

Community psychiatry includes a consciousness of the fact that one is modeling ego behavior on a slightly larger stage and *all the time.*

If a clinician is observed speaking impatiently or disrespectfully to a receptionist or a janitor, it will not matter how skillful or sensitive he or she is with the patient. The patient will always identify with the one who is demeaned.

If, on the other hand, there is an air of reciprocity and mutuality, perhaps even a hint of equality in the way people speak to one another, there is an immediate, inescapable therapeutic effect even before the patient is asked into the private space of the clinician.

Waiting is the essence of the here and now, an existential moment in which learning can take place through a suspended consciousness. There may be nothing more important to the person waiting than to become aware, as if from the corner of one's eye, that there is a consciousness of community around one. The waiting room of a clinic is more revealing of its potential for help than its interviewing rooms. "Waiting *is,*" somebody once wrote. It is the moment around which anticipation, anxiety, and longing pivot.

In the clinic, as in the community, it is in the micro-behaviors, the details, in which therapy resides. It is the music of a voice that conveys its emotional meaning, and music is in the intervals as much as in the notes. One can ask, "How are you doing?" in as many different ways as there are answers, and to a large degree the answer is predetermined by the way the question is put. This is not a mere nicety. It can be a matter of life and death.

The way one asks if someone is thinking about suicide largely preordains the response. When someone is asked his or her name, it usually does not matter whether the setting is a law court, kindergarten class, or dating bar. But the question "Are you thinking of ending your life?" is much more complex, with dozens of other questions buried within it: "Do you trust me?" "Are you determined to die no matter what?" "Does part of you want to live?" "Is it really death you want or to change something in your life?" "What do you feel so guilty or ashamed about?" "Are you angry?" "Why now?" "Do you trust me?" . . . .

This is a confidence game with very high stakes, higher, of course, for the patient than the therapist, but not meaningless for him or her. When a patient commits suicide after one last conflicted appeal for help or understanding, when the last delicate thread of contact with the world is snapped and the clinician is left holding a limp fragment, the sense of defeat that results is from not a technical failure but a human one. It is a failure of community.

The particular responsibility of a community psychiatrist is to be the symbol or manifestation or one of the bearers of what is left of our connectedness to one another. It is a mark of the decadence of our society that this connectedness has been so completely professionalized.

But as long as it existed as a profession, community psychiatry had a quality of immanence. A chance encounter in the street or indirect ones in the clinic had the same effect as a drug prescription or a psychotherapeutic interpretation. And now community psychiatry is gone.

FIVE

Mine only appears to be a hard-hat job. In fact, considering that I spend my life with the distillate of madness, it turns out to be among the safer jobs in the world, which may be more a comment on sanity than the nature of my work.

I often remind my coworkers that our patients are moved to violence only when they are disdained, denigrated, or ignored. As long as they are treated with respect, it does not seem to matter how impulse-ridden, paranoid, or powerful they are. And while paranoids may be deluded about everybody else in the world, it is rare for them to be suspicious of their own therapists. They do not have to be, because to the extent that the therapist sits and listens, i.e., takes him or her seriously, the paranoid person does not have to rely on the desperate extremities of exhausted narcissism to prove that he or she exists. The patient is not as invisible to the therapist as he or she feels to the rest of the world.

Such psychodynamic wisdom is not always accepted by my colleagues. Newcomers to mental health professionalism insist for a while on the simple tautological truth: "Crazy is crazy."

Nor is it only the ingenuous who are scared of psychotics. Many seasoned psychoanalysts would not touch such a patient "with a ten-foot pole."

One multiply analyzed professor emeritus during his tenure as superintendent of a mental hospital was known to carry a gun. He came out of the West and affected a saloon-door swagger, but confided to a colleague that his back-pocket pistol was obtained in his adult eastern days, because "you never know how some schizophrenic might react to a cut in his ward privileges." To my knowledge, while there were many such cuts, never did the bad-hat professor have to whip out his derringer and step over the chastened, bullet-ridden body of a patient while blowing the smoke from the barrel as he sauntered on to his next appointment.

One occasionally hears that a "former mental patient" has gone on a rampage and shot some innocent people at a shopping mall. The press is properly outraged, as they always are by random acts of individual violence. (Systemic violence is more acceptable.) The first questions asked after such an event include "Was the perpetrator ever mentally ill?" and "Whose patient was he?"

There have been occasional instances in a mental hospital or a clinic when a patient has killed a clinician or two, but banks, post offices, and fast-food outlets seem to have had more than their share of shootings. There seems to be no completely safe place to work or even to stay at home in this gun-toting culture, in which the right to bear arms is sacred as long as they are not used for the purpose of rebellion.

Nevertheless, rare though it may be, the killing of a clinician induces one to quickly review one's own patients and reflect back on those who are, have ever been, or might possibly become violent.

Mania is the major problem. I remember one woman who was ordinarily depressed, barely audible, and almost invisible. Her daughter called me to the house, begging me to hospitalize her mother because she was acting "crazy." When I got there, my chronically depressed patient, ordinarily as unprepossessing as a wraith of smoke, had become transformed into at least three of the Furies. She flailed at me with her cigarette-clenching fist so that I received a slight burn on my cheek and my glasses were flung from their perch before I could back out of the apartment. She followed me to the street, having shed her bathrobe, and caught the attention of passersby by shouting imprecations.

As often happens, once she was securely tied to an ambulance stretcher, she calmed down, and by the time she got to the hospital, she was so controlled that I had a hard time convincing the on-call resident that she needed to be admitted.

After she was salted down with Lithium, she reverted to her depressed baseline and, interestingly, forgot about her street demonstration. She actually recalled and apologized for her behavior several years later as she was getting "high" again. She had gone without sleep for several days, and along with a few uncharacteristic wisecracks, she suddenly remembered with a giggle having thrown off her clothes and presenting her screaming self to the people of Chelsea.

Ambulance attendants who are called to transport psychiatric patients often make up for their lack of social skills by strong-arming patients into restraints. I am generally asked to write "restraints *P.R.N.* (as needed)" on commitment papers to give them the legal justification for doing so, "just in case." But every once in a while, they ask for the police as well, particularly when the patient is as big as he or she is unmotivated.

Once I was called by the police themselves. A middle-aged man was locked in his apartment, threatening to use a shotgun on somebody unnamed. Since he hadn't actually committed a crime, the police thought "the shrink" might cut through some of the due-process details that burdened them, preventing them from locking him up.

They were already there when I arrived at the apartment. One feels a certain inexplicable reassurance in the presence of uniforms when having to confront the less-organized possibilities of violence, as if centuries of centurions, crusaders, conquistadors, and contras had not taught us that order can be more murderous than chaos. I reached the door with an armed escort, feeling a peculiar mixture of privilege and foolishness, which immediately dissipated when the officers arranged themselves, dragnet-style, on either side of me, and unbuttoned their holsters. With me standing directly in front of it, one of the officers banged on the door with his sideways extended fist and shouted, "It's all right, Jim. We're sending in the doctor."

I gave him a Steve Martin look of twisted quizzicality and stage-whispered, "Are you nuts? I'm not going in there!"

The psychiatrist asking "Are you nuts?" struck the appropriate note with the officer in charge, who figured out what I meant. "You want us to go in there with you?"

"I want you to go in first, and if everything is okay, then maybe I'll come in."

Maybe he, too, had read the Rex Morgan, M.D., comic strip that I remembered from many years before, in which charismatic Rex walks past the police barricade into the house with the maniac, convinces him to hand over the gun, and walks him out to the waiting ambulance with a hand on the guy's shoulder. I remembered the comic strip but was not ready to follow it to the letter.

The law went in first, ascertained that there was, in fact, no shotgun in evidence, and invited me in to decide whether or not this deluded, hallucinating, psychotic man needed to return to the asylum. He was perfectly agreeable to going to the hospital, but as he was about to walk out to the waiting ambulance with nobody's arm around his shoulder, he suddenly stopped and said, "Wait a minute," and scuttled into the bedroom.

The movie I was watching had him dragging out his Uzi and mowing down everything in sight. I didn't want to sound like Kojak growling orders to the boys, so I decided to follow him just to make sure his movie wasn't the same as mine.

I watched him bend down to the side of the bed. "This is it," I said to myself. Here I am on the front page of the *Boston Herald*: "SHRINK SHOT DEAD BY FORMER MENTAL PATIENT AS COPS LOOK ON." I was about to shout something incoherent to the cops when Jim methodically lined up the front toes of his leather slippers and then, with a sigh of satisfaction, straightened up to walk out with us. It was, at the same moment, an image of charming domesticity and chillingly psychotic obsessionalism.

He was discharged not long afterward, and a couple of years later I pronounced him dead when his wife called the clinic to say that she thought he had committed suicide. It was the same location, but different cops. His wife, separated but friendly to him and living in an adjacent apartment, had not heard from him in some time. He did not answer the door or the phone, so she called the police and her therapist at the clinic, who asked me to to go in with her. We arrived as the police were breaking down the now familiar door.

And for years after, his wife went around threatening to kill people, including, from time to time, me.

But threats against me were not unusual. One source was a Cuban émigré, an aging, dandified, antirevolutionary alcoholic, who did not have the resources or initiative to leave the island in 1959 and waited until two decades later for the Mariel boat lift.

He would not keep appointments, but Alfredo would walk in to the clinic in his polished white shoes, reeking of rum, swearing to his prerevolutionary gods that he had not *tomado nada*, and demanding sleep medicine.

Sleep medicine is a contradiction in terms. Wakefulness is not a disease curable by medication. Shakespeare's "Sweet, oblivious antidotes" to the perturbations of life, like narcotics for its sharper edges, do not restore the troubled sleepless to a natural condition. Sleep is a giving up of sorts, a trusting to the night, and the hypervigilant, the guilt-ridden, and the already intoxicated cannot expect a warranty for sleep on demand.

Pills offering such a promise are available, however, and while there are hangovers, amnesia, irritability, and overt addictions among its costs, and the sleep which they provide is not the same as that which comes unaided, they can be prescribed and purchased. Indeed, the one thing most often requested by patients when asked by the feckless physician, "What can I do for you?" is sleeping "medication."

Alfredo demanded it. He felt it was his right as a refugee from communism, and was indifferent to my sanctimonious speeches about sleep rendered in splintered Spanish.

Sometimes, to get rid of him, I gave him a prescription for a common antihistamine, which, couched in its generic, chemical-sounding name, seems to have more pharmacological presence than its over-the-counter sib.

Alcohol is not a good sedative because it is too quickly metabolized, and a few short hours after its bedtime administration, the patient is wide awake with the sparkling intensity which, at the more remote outposts of alcoholism, will become the frank D.T.'s.

Alfredo would drink himself into a stupor watching the *novelas* on TV and would awaken at 3 a.m. with a mixture of longing for the crumbling pastels of *La Habana Vieja* and terror that the Chelsea police might suddenly become as intrusive as the Committee for the Defense of the Revolution.

Some years before, he had presented his importunate self to a clinic colleague who, on learning that Alfredo was Cuban, thought to establish a more cordial relationship by revealing that he, the clinician, had recently visited Cuba. Alfredo, in a paranoid, alcoholic, antirevolutionary panic ran screaming from the clinic in fear that the confused, shamefaced therapist would consult with Raul or Fidel about how to get him back to the prison on the Isle of Pines.

This *contretemps* did not prevent him from returning later with more demands for a sedative, though he made plain to the receptionist that never again would he have anything to do with the communist on the staff.

My own more politically neutral ministrations were not particularly appreciated. Once after I refused to give him anything stronger for sleep than the Benadryl whose potency in its generic form he was beginning to doubt, he announced that he was going to get a gun and kill me.

I suppose a scrupulous and prudent psychiatrist would have warned the intended victim in accordance with the Tarasoff Decision, contacted the police in the jurisdiction in which the intended victim resided, and instituted involuntary hospitalization proceedings. These are the appropriate steps to be taken when a patient threatens homicide, in dereliction of which a therapist could be liable for a malpractice suit. I wondered if my wife and children were so mercenary as to sue me for malpractice when I was the murder victim. As to calling the suburban police department where I resided to tell them that an Hispanic man had threatened to kill one of the town's white, middle-class, professional residents, I somehow doubted this would contribute to a reduction in the world's burden of racial hatred. I could have signed a pink paper and sent the Chelsea police after him, but he had been in and out of inpatient psychiatric units many times and would have been back on the streets in a few days anyway.

The next day he was back, having forgotten that he threatened to kill me, and a little embarrassed when I reminded him, but not so much so that he was not ready to ask once again for a sleeping pill.

According to Emerson, a foolish consistency is the hobgoblin of small minds. Large-minded, Alfredo came to the clinic some time later, again drunk, shouting at me that he was going to kill me because all the medicine for sleep I had given him over the years had caused him to become sexually impotent. He would not hear my professional opinion that alcohol might have had more to do with it (or my unstated, nonprofessional one that counterrevolutionaries are often doomed to impotence). He stormed out, once again vowing to get a gun.

A few days later, he came back asking for pills for impotence, which I indicated I did not have. Later still, I was called by a urologist who, moved by the romantic failures of this anticommunist, was on the verge of inserting a prosthesis. I suggested that Alfredo might not be the best candidate for a permanent erection but did not add that if the thing should not make him irresistible to every woman in Chelsea, Alfredo might threaten to shoot *him*. Doctors who provide artificial erections have to look out for themselves.

I seem to have a high tolerance to murder threats. Another of my patients, a fixture in Chelsea, would greet me on the street from a distance of a half block or more with shouts at the top of his lungs about my imminent demise at the hands of the Mafia or the Hell's Angels. "They're coming to get you," he would scream. My casual smile and wave back must have been as confusing to onlookers as the threats themselves.

Nevertheless, I *was* once assaulted. I was sucker-punched in my office. It was not a bad punch; it was "pulled," revealing the ambivalence of the throw. I was more astonished by its source than its occurrence.

Arnold was another well-known resident of Chelsea, a young man who had shown promise as an artist in high school, but whose career and life were blighted by a combination of alcohol and psychosis that induced him to take occasional swings at such targets as cops and stop signs. His art was just as irrepressible, and manifested itself on various billboards whose Coke and Camel messages were whited out and replaced by Motif #1. He wielded a rather sentimental palette, with lots of pink in the clouds, sea, and sand.

I had one of his canvases in the office. It was not really a gift. He had said that it could hang there in case someone wanted to buy it. And while it has had many admirers, most of them quite mad, there have been no offers, so over the years it had come to belong there. Arnold would glance at it when he came by for his monthly prescription for tranquilizers. With the instinct of the artist who is never quite done with the work, he would occasionally wander over to add a bit more pink here or there.

I encourage everyone to be creative and tend to be very appreciative of every artistic production. To people who say, "I can't draw," or, "I don't know how to write poetry," I insist that they at least try. I remind them that every member of an Australian aboriginal tribe has the responsibility for decorating his or her shield or pot. Some indeed may be better decorated than others, but that does not matter. Being a member of the community means being an artist.

But in non-tribal Chelsea, the other side of the "I can't do it" coin tends to emerge once someone has been induced to draw a picture or write a fragment of verse. The question becomes "Do you think I can sell it?" If anything is worth anything in that shattered market society, then it must be worth money. So like a muse suddenly turning cheap, I try to seduce people into the arts and discourage any expectation of a payoff.

Arnold said he was a "painter" and not yet an "artist," until he drank or smoked dope and became paranoid, when such finely tuned judgments were blurred.

I had just returned from a vacation. I was sitting at my desk writing a note, when suddenly I felt a punch on the right side of my jaw. Arnold was standing there red-faced and trembling.

"What the hell is the matter with you?" I asked.

"I got evicted while you were on vacation. I lost all my art materials. It wouldn't have happened if you were here. You better send me to the hospital."

"You bet," I said. Later, he apologized and we continued on friendly terms. And while people would see us occasionally walking down the street together and everybody still treats him well, he now carries the reputation as "the only guy in Chelsea who ever hit the Doc." I think he feels good about it.

There is an uglier form of violence in Chelsea and similar places. The combination of density, racism, poverty, and youth equals mayhem. Shakespeare, as always, had an understanding of this relationship and, as always, one has to pay attention to the side action in his plays to hear his voice.

There are two unnamed murderers in *Macbeth*. When the crazed king's paranoia begins to feed on itself, he calls them in and offers them a deal that is difficult to refuse. In response, one of them says:

I am one, my liege, who has been so incensed by the vile blows and buffets of the world that I am reckless what I do to spite it.

The other adds:

And I am so weary with disaster, tugged by fortune that I would set my life on any chance to mend it or be rid of it.

Poverty causes murder through angry indifference and desperate opportunism. The young people of Chelsea look around and realize what is in store for them: a trap. The middle class makes a deal with life. We feel a sense of control over the course of events because we define them. We make a Pascal's bet to give up the moment, to put a leash on lust and rage on the chance that the future will pay us back with interest. The really rich, of course, do not need to bother with Pascal's odds. They can indulge the here and now and keep their futures intact.

But the poor are powerless. To them, the future is a foreign world. Jerome Kagan's observations of child development in different cultures led him to conclude that social class is the implacable predictor of an individual's sense of mastery over events. When a child learns as early as six that he or she is the plaything of destiny, that external forces determine one's security and satisfaction, that one is helpless to redirect the smallest eddy in the stream of time, then there is no sense of purpose and no capacity to think of the future.

Powerlessness is the final common path of urban poverty, regardless of culture. Martin Seligman's concept of "learned helplessness" describes the process of internalizing that powerlessness. The more one is exposed to events over which one has no control, the more one is convinced that there is no way to control anything. Finding over and over again that things happen *to* her rather than being directed *by* her, a young woman in poverty begins to feel that even those things that are actually in her control are beyond her, such as the ability to soothe a distressed infant.

One of the characteristics of a life of poverty is an increased frequency of life events. The studies of Brown, Wing, and Birely at the Maudsley Hospital in England have demonstrated that during the six weeks before a psychotic episode, more events have happened in the lives of patients than during other periods or during the same period in the lives of matched non-patients.

This is particularly the case in so-called "high emotional expressive" families, in which the affective ripples after each event are amplified rather than muted. As an additional and independent feature, the psychotic patient is characterized by his or her inability to withdraw from that arena of intensified affect. There are no retreats, no doors to close, there is no personal life space, so that the very lack of privacy for the stressed individual becomes itself a major stressor.

Being trapped in an environment of intensified affect surrounding an increased frequency of events is pathological. This describes the violent life of the young in Chelsea, with its endless sequence of fires, accidents, illnesses, job losses, pregnancies, marriages, divorces, births, deaths; hardly has a person recovered from one wave of change than another comes along.

Calhoun's studies of the effects of social density on the behavior of animals found that there is a refractory period after every encounter, from a courtship approach by a friendly animal to an aggressive one by a predator. During this period, *any* subsequent encounter is experienced as aggressive.

The more encounters one has, the greater the percentage of negative encounters one experiences. The density and velocity of adverse life events in the face of their helplessness leaves the young in Chelsea with a sense of endless abrasiveness.

Erich Fromm has written, "Destructiveness is the outcome of unlived life." The less consequence there is to a life, the more it is squandered. The Centers for Disease Control reported that homicide among African-American males aged 15 to 24 increased by 67 percent between 1984 and 1988 and is now their leading cause of death. When an economy crumbles, it falls faster at the bottom than at the top, and ours is a society that is closing schools and opening prisons.

Violence feeds on itself. The more there is, the more there will be. Dr. Freud was wrong about this. There is not a constitutionally endowed reservoir of aggressive energy in each individual that must be released or it festers into neuroticism. In fact, the more that anger is expressed, the more it is experienced. Football players manifest more violent and aggressive imagery on Rorschach tests after a scrimmage than before. Every expression of rage can be kindling for another.

The mind is as much a social as a neurological structure. Our mental life resides within the relationship between society and the individual nervous system, and both mental illness and violence are disruptions of that relationship. Disruption can take place anywhere along the social-neurological spectrum of mind; its moorings can be torn at either end.

Social as well as neurological forces can cause a level of arousal at which every additional stimulus requires less intensity than the one before to produce a convulsion. Mob violence has its own dynamics, so that people with relatively ordinary nervous systems can become transformed into explosive, rampaging packs of bestiality.

On the other hand, some people have compromised nervous systems, one feature of which is the inability to filter and select stimuli and respond in a controlled and functional way. For example, the cerebral cortex, the place where rationality and civility are rooted, is an inhibiting agency. Damage to the cerebral cortex results in a convulsion, an unrestrained firing of neurons, a nonselective, uncontrollable, and often destructive response to a minimal stimulus.

The individual act of violence is not the same as a convulsion; murder may be a rational, planned, and systematic business. But the propensity to violence, the too quick and easy resort to it, at times reflects a nervous system that has been damaged.

Poverty is damaging in many different ways. One of these is in its effects on the individual nervous system as a result of compromised reproductive health. This was one of the currents of devastation I learned about in crossing the larger whirlpool of poverty itself.

There is a trap in such an inquiry. It is the trap into which contemporary psychiatry and social science may yet fall before recognizing it as the very one engineered by Nazi medicine during another of this century's dark moments.

To identify a neurological dimension to individual violence must not lead to a public policy preoccupation with the individual manifestation of such defects but to an exploration of their shared and social origins.

Early in 1992, consistent with the times and the ideology of the administration that appointed him, the director of the National Institute of Mental Health commented that his agency would attempt to illuminate urban violence through a search for "biological markers." By age five, a child (most likely poor and black) could be identified as a future perpetrator of violence and a preventive intervention attempted.

This represented a reprise of the research done on prisoners a generation ago that attempted to relate an extra Y chromosome to criminality. And it shared in the tradition of Astin's research on "protest-prone students" and the suggestion made by several psychiatrists during the civil disorders of the sixties that riot participants might be suffering from temporal lobe epilepsy. Every rebirth of fascism will rely on such group predictors of behavior as the most implacable form of social control.

The history of technology has always been characterized by the invention of hammers and the subsequent search for heads to bang with them. When I, therefore, raise the question of an exploration into the role of reproductive health in mental illness and violence, I run the risk of running my fingers along the stainless steel bars of that trap. The focus must be on poverty, not its victims. It is as a measure of social injustice that we have to count rates of prematurity and other adversities of pregnancy, not as a means of predicting the deviance or dysfunction of the human beings who suffer from them.

SIX

For all we know, guns may have nothing whatsoever to do with revolution. We must see to it that children are born properly. This is real revolution, of this I am quite sure.

Isaac Babel, *The Palace of Motherhood*, 1918

On Saturday, October 5, 1991, a filler appeared at the bottom of the front page of the *New York Times*. Headlined, "Poverty's Toll on Health Is Plague of U.S. Schools," it was not really "news" in the journalistic sense but rather one of those references to an ongoing current in contemporary life.

The article referred to a ghetto school in Pittsburgh in which teachers struggle to teach children whose subtle neurological impairments interfere with their sight or hearing or their capacity to calm themselves when upset. The article related school failure to the fact that 13 percent of the children attending the school were born underweight.

The overall rate of low birth weight in America is 6.9 percent, about the same as in Bulgaria. Even when apparently "normal" in intelligence or motor development, a large number of these children will have behavioral or learning problems in school, problems that will foreclose their education or even the possibility of their being adequately socialized.

In Chelsea, the major reason children were referred to the clinic for treatment was "school problems." This did not refer to such vague learning difficulties as dyslexia. In Chelsea, the learning problems were more gross and obvious: children who could not sit still for more than a few minutes, frustration levels so low that screaming tantrums were provoked by the slightest effort to set limits, rage reactions so intense that other children were terrorized, an incapacity to learn to read at all.

Some years ago, two investigators, Birch and Gussow, wrote: "Of all the human complications of pregnancy and parturition, no single condition is more clearly associated with a wide range of insults to the nervous system than too early expulsion into the world. . . ." The brain is so complex and critical an organ that its development begins earliest and ends latest, not being complete until months after actual birth. A premature birth sends that vulnerable, developing network into the harsh light and crashing sounds of extrauterine existence before all its tracks have been laid down and wires fully lined.

Birch and Gussow found four times the rate of impaired hearing among premature children as compared to matched controls. In addition, 59 percent of the premature children had visual disturbances.

The measurement of intelligence has always been marked by racial, gender, and class bias. The I.Q. test, whatever else it is, serves as a rough predictor of school performance, if only because the tasks measured by the test are the same tasks taught in school—mainly the manipulation of words. The bias is in the choice of the words tested, so that the intelligence of white middle-class children is never challenged by asking them to distinguish a *tostada* from a *tostina*, or *running a game* from *playing the dozens*. However, in general, low birth weight exerts an effect on intelligence as measured by the I.Q. test. Middle- and upper-class children are better protected from this effect than the poor. The advantages of material security and comfort seem to compensate almost fully for the risks of low birth weight.

On the other hand, there is a disturbing lack of correlation between I.Q. and school performance among low-birth-weight children. Birch and Gussow found that of 36 premature children who tested with normal I.Q.s, 20 had difficulties in school, with 11 having to repeat one or more of the first three grades.

To a large extent, prematurity or low birth weight is a function of poverty. As with mental illness, there is a direct relationship between social class and average birth weight. The frequency of children born prematurely to African-American women is twice as high as for whites, the difference explainable by poverty. There is no genetic or inherent reason for black babies to be born sooner and smaller than white ones.

What is it about poverty that results in small babies with compromised nervous systems? One factor that can be teased out of this whirlpool of destruction has to do with the mother's age. This makes me think about Ellie.

She was not my patient. Her own mother was—a chronically depressed, bedridden woman paralyzed by multiple sclerosis. For four years, I made weekly home visits to Victoria, who was referred to me after a serious suicide attempt. Victoria and her common-law husband Larry, Ellie's father, owned one of those nickel-and-dime variety stores, a "spa," as it was called in Chelsea, where cigarettes, soda, lottery tickets, and candy were sold from early morning to late at night every day of the week. It was a social institution as much as an enterprise, as people hung around to talk while Vicky kept a watchful, if tolerant, eye on the children whose pennies did not quite add up to the cost of a candy bar. Children got no credit at "Vicky's," but the police were rarely called for the frequently attempted micro-thefts.

Her illness rapidly progressed so that Vicky was soon unable to attend to the store, even from a wheelchair, and eventually her husband gave up his manual labor job to run the store himself.

The store did not thrive under his hands. The profit margin of such an establishment is so thin that it barely matches the salary of an entry-level job. The distributors of Coke and Pepsi do not like to deliver relatively small volumes of canned soda to such stores and discount so heavily their deliveries to supermarket chains that it was sometimes cheaper for "Vicky's" to get its soda from the supermarket than from the distributor.

Vicky tried to manage the store from her bed, but Larry, a burly ex-Marine, complained that *he* now had to make the decisions, and his resentment of her illness took the form of complaining about her efforts to control the store when she wasn't there. She became paranoid about money, and before long, paranoid about the many single women ("douche bags," as she called them) who would stop by the store. As it later turned out, Larry was indeed sleeping around, but Vicky's paranoia, the projection of her helplessness and rage at her own body, resulted in furious fights even before her fears became true. Lying in bed, she would scream out and strike him with all her feeble power. Once she scratched him and he hit her back. He protested that he only hit her softly—"I could have killed her if I'd really hit her"—but she was bruised for weeks. It was after such a fight that she made her suicide attempt, and she was constantly thereafter shouting that she would swallow all of her (many) pills or leave the gas jets on and then "he can have the store and his douche bags and Ellie, too."

Ellie was nine when I began my visits to the house. Her room was small, barely larger than her bed, separated from the chaotic bedroom of her parents by a thin plywood wall. All the groans of pain and ever less frequently of pleasure came through that wall, and much of my futile effort as a psychiatrist went toward developing in the couple a sense of boundaries and responsibility toward their daughter.

Larry would have to ask a friend to mind the store when he was at home for my visits, so our attempts at regular "couples treatment" were limited. They were mainly efforts to stop their arguments, in any case. "Let him finish and then I'll listen to you." "Try to control your anger and put into words what you want her to know." "Don't raise your voice; we can hear you." "Do you want to respond to what he (she) said?" Such were my interventions.

When I saw Vicky alone, I would tell her that she had to stop making suicide threats if she cared about her daughter. While not consistent with a psychodynamic approach to suicide prevention, such statements got her attention and eventually worked. However, for years Ellie saw it as her own responsibility to keep her mother alive. Coming home from school, she would count her mother's remaining pills and check the gas jets before she threw down her books. It was, she said, the hardest part of her day, the scariest. The fights were also bad, but not as bad as rushing home worrying whether Vicky were alive or dead.

My conversations with Ellie were always over her shoulder. She never really wanted to talk to me and refused my suggestion that she come to the clinic to see if one of the "big sister"-like counselors there could help her. She saw therapy as something for people like her mother, and was possessive of any free time. She would take advantage of my weekly presence to spend an hour with a friend before hurrying back to make supper.

Ellie was a bright, adorable nine-year-old with wide and worrying eyes. Apparently she was getting A's from the nuns at the St. Rose School, but they complained on report cards about her being preoccupied and distracted. Too much of life was forcing itself too soon on the delicate filigree of her preadolescent mind. I would sometimes hear her hum along to "golden oldies" in perfect harmony like a small silver bell. Her drawings of unicorns were lively and colorful: irresistible colts with fierce, fictive weapons coming from their heads.

Once I asked, "Ellie, do you ever think about your future?"

A shrug. "No."

"You're very smart. You could go to college."

"I'm not going to college. I'm going to get a job."

“But if you stay in school and go to college, you could get a better job. You can do anything.”

“I’m not that smart.”

“You’re very smart. College would be easy for you. And there are scholarships to make it free. Don’t you ever have dreams about what grown-up life could possibly be?”

“Yes, I have a dream.”

“Well?”

“I could never do it.”

“Tell me.”

“I could never do it.” There was a long pause. “I dream of being a secretary.”

This was her sense of the vast, inaccessible world of middle-class life, the TV world of a secretary, with its bogus glitz and badinage and modest, modern apartments overlooking the city and charming, successful men wanting to marry her: all that irresistible mythology, as false and dreamlike and unattainable as a unicorn. Such was the hidden injury of her class that the polished image of a clerical functionary at the lowest level of that world out there—*across the bridge*—felt impossible. Her future in her mind would more likely be spent in factories or, as it turned out, pregnancies and welfare. That was a future she could create for herself, and she began its creation four years later, at the age of 13.

Thirteen-year-old children having children is not a shocking affair in Chelsea. It is a mundane event. The reactions of their mothers vary. Many groan in despair at the entrapment of their little girls, who before their eyes become transformed into prematurely ripe, and all too soon, like themselves, prematurely aged women. But many others accept it as a matter of course. Only about a third of the quarter of a million women under age 17 in this country who become pregnant choose abortion. Only about five percent of the children born to teenagers are placed for adoption. By and large, these children born to children are raised by the children themselves or their own exhausted mothers.

The prevailing attitude in Chelsea, especially among Hispanic families, is that the shame of a teenage daughter’s pregnancy can be erased by her marriage. So, often enough, the child with a child marries another child. Subsequent pregnancies soon occur and, as the majority of teenage marriages end in divorce or abandonment, the result is an impoverished, lonely, overwhelmed, dependent girl with several infants. The younger she was at her first pregnancy, the more children she is likely to have, and the more closely spaced they are likely to be.

Women under 17 have a higher rate of all complications of pregnancy—anemia, toxemia of pregnancy, urinary tract infections, uterine dysfunction, inadequate pelvic size, and premature rupture of the placenta. Each of these complications threatens the health and neurological competence of the infant and increases the likelihood of an infant born too small or too soon with a higher probability of having emotional and intellectual handicaps.

The mortality rate for these infants is three to five times greater than for others, and the survivors are more dependent, distractible, overactive, hostile, and impulsive than matched controls. They are very difficult children, born to women whose capacities for care may be very limited. And while it is certainly true that the official reports of child abuse and neglect disproportionately focus on the poor and minorities for behaviors that are ignored among white, middle-class parents, it seems inescapably true that having a child before the age of 20, alone and living in poverty, stresses many young mothers to the point that they may be abusive or neglectful.

Life is a voyage on a river without shores. Living an impoverished life is like traveling in a small and weak vessel on turbulent waters. Pregnancy is a narrowing of the river, a channeling of its force and momentum, a cascade. The influences of poverty on birth exist long before the pregnancy, endure throughout life, and are passed on. A mother's poor health, for example, may result from her own compromised birth, inadequate health care, exposure to pathogens, and deficient diet—which she carried throughout her own life and which become more severe, more concentrated, and more consequential during pregnancy.

The higher population destiny of poor urban areas results in more contact with bacteria and viruses than in middle-class communities. Poor nutrition results in a lowered resistance to infection, so that when exposed to the same streptococci, tubercle bacilli, or viruses as others, a poor woman is more likely to develop rheumatic fever, glomerulonephritis, tuberculosis, or influenza. A greater frequency of infections results in a greater use of antibiotics, with associated allergic reactions, resistant organisms, and secondary infections. And the residues of antibiotics in the intestines affect bacteria necessary for the absorption of amino acids. This results in even poorer nutrition, with yet lower levels of gamma globulin and yet lower resistance to infection. The whirlpool grows wider.

Calcium and iron deficiencies in the diets of the poor increase the absorption and toxicity of lead and other toxins from the environment. At the same time, there are greater numbers and higher concentrations of such poisons in low-income neighborhoods.

These vicious circles in the river of life become devastating during pregnancy. The damage sustained accumulates through life, leaving an even more destructive legacy to subsequent generations of children. The river becomes a rapid.

The extent of anemia found among low-income children ranges from 28 percent to 80 percent, depending on the study. Anemia results in intellectual deficiency, lassitude, emotional irritability, and depression, as well as a greater vulnerability to lead poisoning, which itself causes behavioral problems and learning difficulties. Lead passes completely through the placenta and concentrates in the developing nervous system of the already-compromised fetus, so each subsequent generation is more lead-poisoned than the one before. And lead poisoning in turn results in anemia, with still greater vulnerability to lead exposure, completing the vicious circle.

Vitamin C, calcium, and riboflavin deficiencies result in lowered resistance to infections. When children have sore throats or colds or ear infections, they often eat even less nutritious diets than usual, so yet another whirlpool of pathology results.

One study of low-income 10- to 13-year-old children in New York found that 71 percent had inadequate diets. All too soon these children will be parents, with yet another generation swept up in the whirlpools within whirlpools of lives of malnutrition, infection, and lead poisoning.

And there is more smoking, obesity, and hypertension among the poor. These complicate pregnancy and lead to cardiopulmonary diseases and diabetes, which also complicate pregnancy. The medications used to treat these conditions and the many other ailments of the poor are often themselves teratogenic, i.e., negatively affect the developing fetus.

It remains a question whether maternal and child health is more compromised by street drugs or by the legal ones prescribed by physicians and sold over the counter. But the combination of substances used and abused and the ill health and unhealthy living for which they are taken adds to the cascade of disease. Each pregnancy among the poor seems to distill and pass on to the following generation the ill health of previous ones with growing ferocity.

In Chelsea, I would sometimes feel like the little Dutch boy trying to plug hole after hole with fingers too small and too few. At times my sense of desperation spilled out on the families I was trying to help, finding myself trying to intimidate them into empowerment, making them feel guilty for being victims. They were all too ready to blame themselves for their misery and were expert at living with guilt.

I became involved with the DeAngelo family when their ten-year-old boy, one of four children, was found playing with matches after having been the cause of a fire that had burned them out of their previous apartment. I started treating Stevie alone, like a technician. I had done some reading and consulted an expert about fire-setting children and decided to use the "exhaustion technique" to stop what is obviously a symptom of troubled emotions, but a symptom that must be controlled.

The technique consists of placing a box of kitchen matches before the child and having him light one after another until the novelty wears off. The child becomes bored and fretful and wants to stop, but the rule is that he cannot stop before the whole box is used up. The same thing is done for another session and then a third. Anecdotal case reports reveal a high success rate in stopping children from playing with matches when the three sessions are completed.

I gave up midway during the second session. I was not enough of a behaviorist to endure Stevie's tears. He whimpered at first, then sobbed, and finally wept openly because he could not stand it anymore. We stopped and went back to drawing pictures, which, for him, were wild and chaotic exercises involving monsters and houses surrounded by a barrage of colored lines not unlike fire. The children in his houses were frail stick figures; the parents were bulbous, inert masses.

I began visiting the family at home, the small second floor of a ramshackle house on a vast empty lot next to a busy highway. It was one of those lonely houses near a fast road, seen but unremarked by thousands of people rushing by every day. The children had to walk along the highway for several hundred feet in order to get to sidewalks that would take them a half dozen blocks further to school. This daily engagement with predatory traffic preyed constantly on the minds of the parents. Indeed, one of the other children was hit by a car and sustained a broken bone, fortunately not a head injury, during their tenure "on the parkway."

There is a peculiar subterranean ambivalence about car injuries in Chelsea. The streets being playgrounds, parents live in constant fear of the sounds of shrieking brakes. But there is, on the other hand, a lottery mentality about such accidents as about everything else in low-income life. A "settlement" for a small injury can help people out of debt or remove the nagging, guilt-ridden sense of a deficient "spirit of Christmas." Money is always on the minds of the poor, and too many families in Chelsea are waiting for the interminable turns of the ratchet wheels of law courts to provide them with the bonus that comes with a broken bone, or worse. The lawyers, of course, get most of it.

Ms. DeAngelo was a massive woman, always at the kitchen table, always smoking, always playing solitaire. She accepted my visits with the same indifference that she accepted the other catastrophes of life. I was

merely another of a long series of butting-in agency people who judged and tried to control her behavior in the name of "help."

Her husband was a small, practically invisible wraith of a man, a factory worker away at work most of the time at a company that manufactured chemicals. There was a perpetual smell about him, something sweet and volatile—benzene, toluene, or acetone. I was later involved with a strike at his plant because the owners refused to acknowledge that these were hazardous substances and would not provide masks and gloves to the workers. But that was years later. At that time, I merely noted as another source of stress that when this short, thin man looking like an underexposed 35-mm slide with too little light behind it, like a mere extension of his own cigarette smoke, walked into the room, his wife and two of his children began wheezing from chronic asthma.

Cigarette smoke was everywhere. Automobile fumes were everywhere. The smell of volatile chemicals from Charlie's clothes was everywhere. Behind the house was an auto junkyard where there were frequent fires, usually involving tires and lead batteries.

Every time I left the house, it was with a headache. I could never tell whether it was from the noxious, nauseating mix of vapors in the air or frustration at what I was doing there.

There was no place else for them to live. Once they were short of money and were threatened with eviction. Wondering what my first supervisor in psychotherapy, an analyst of the old school sniffing like a beagle for signs of countertransference, would have said, I wrote out a check for $60 and handed it to Ms. DeAngelo. She hoped she wouldn't have to use it, but took it matter-of-factly.

Maybe I assumed that I now had the right to nag a little. I finally began suggesting that if the adults didn't smoke, there wouldn't be so many matches around the house. This was ignored.

The children did not look well. They had a pale, pasty look to their chubbiness. When I glanced into the refrigerator, I saw only Pepsi bottles and peanut butter and luncheon meats. There was always candy on the table. The TV set was always on and the children reached for M&M's from the table with the same habitual joylessness, the same lassitude, the same sense of velleity, as their mother reached for a cigarette. These were pleasures so ground down, so worn thin by indulgence, so bearing the weight of otherwise empty lives that they were only the rumpled wrappers of pleasure, the discarded skins, the bare and barely conscious memory of what was once enjoyed, like the stained finger of a heavy smoker flicking at a cigarette no longer there.

We were on a first-name basis. The younger kids would run in and out shouting, "Hi, Matt," in unison and giggle. Occasionally, one would climb on my lap. Stevie, ever mindful of the exhaustion sessions, kept his distance. While he couldn't call me "Matt" because I had played so complex and authoritarian a role with him, he was too proud to call me "Dr. Dumont" when his contemptible younger siblings were using the familiar, so he called me nothing.

For Marie DeAngelo, it was just "Matt." Perhaps this was a mistake on my part. Maybe I should have left a little of the aura, a touch of the pomp of *Dr.* Silver, the aging, slightly faltering g.p. who gave the kids their shots and bandaged their lacerations, but the psychiatrist who made home visits was "Matt," like a member of the family.

On one occasion, like a member of the family, I "lost it." I had stopped nagging about smoking and stopped offering Nicorette prescriptions and waving my hand at the ambient smoke. She did not *want* to stop smoking, couldn't I understand that? The issue had more or less been laid to rest.

I was sipping tea and Ms. DeAngelo was telling me how much trouble she was having getting the children to come in from the street (the highway) each night for supper. It was always dark by the time they got in, with the rush hour traffic percolating, and she would get hoarse shouting from the window.

An ashtray with a half dozen butts ground and broken like bodies after a disaster was in front of me. The acid stink broke through and knurled behind my eyes. I pushed the ashtray aside. She saw it as the return of my moralizing about her smoking and pushed it back in front of me.

"Goddamnit, Marie," said Matt, the Harvard-trained psychiatrist. "You can be difficult."

She smiled. Did I then apologize, try to explain, return her to the topic? No, I persisted.

"You know, if you were a little more controlled in your own behavior, you might have more control over the kids. You could try to cut down on your smoking. You could drink less Pepsi. You shouldn't talk so much about sex in front of them. You shouldn't have candy on the table all the time. How do you expect the kids to be hungry for supper when they eat candy all day?" My voice rose. The sounds of cartoons came from the other room.

"You should have clear-cut sanctions for the kids." (I said "sanctions.") "If they aren't in by five, no television. They should have tasks around the house. They should do their homework. They shouldn't be out there in the dark. You should control them."

What could she have said? What would *I* have said? Something like: "I didn't ask you to come here and tell me how to run my life. Who do you think you are? Who gave you the right to judge me? Who gave you the sponge to wipe clean the rings on my table? Who gave you the light to shine in the corners of my life? Take your controlled, healthy, smug face, your sympathetic looks, your patience, your glib insight; take your condescending, self-important arrogance out of *my* house and go to hell."

She actually said nothing. She looked at me with a small smile and then blew a long, slow stream of smoke into my face.

I laughed and she laughed. The sounds of cartoons came from the other room.

SEVEN

Mental health consultation is one of the essential features of a community mental health center and the only one to address the issue of prevention. Consultation is easy. Psychotherapy is a little harder. The hardest of all is to be a patient. The farther away you are from the red dirt of human misery, the more comfortable it is, so consultation is relatively easy. Another professional tells you about his or her problems with a client. It isn't *your* problem, and it isn't even your responsibility if something goes wrong based on your advice: it's the supervisor's problem.

In any case, advice with all its presumption of superior knowledge and experience is not the issue, nor is it particularly helpful. People do not want to be told what to do. They want the assurance that they are doing about as well as anyone can, and they want to be understood.

There is within every mental health professional, no matter how mature, well trained, or experienced, a small, dark, locked chamber. Denied, forgotten, or ignored until in an occasional drunken moment or staggering down the wrong street of memory or blundering in the unfamiliar darkness of an insomniac night or buffeted in a sudden emotional squall, it is come upon and flung open. There, a child with a lunatic grin and a shrill mocking laugh sputters out with drool, "Who do you think *you* are?"

The art of mental health consultation is to help a professional to carry on, trying to make things a little easier despite that chamber. The technique is to listen. One asks questions only in part to elicit information or as a guide to what should have been known. Asking questions assures the consultee that one is listening. Since everyone is expecting at any moment to have that hidden room of self-hatred and diffidence discovered, the very fact that the consultant shows a certain patience and respect after listening, and may even seem to understand, is itself the major intervention.

People feel better having been able to put a troublesome situation into words. Kept inside, elbowed by shame and guilt or smeared with self-hatred, it remains murky and sullied. When placed out in the clearer light of social space and found to be tolerated by an "expert," a situation that had been overwhelming suddenly becomes manageable again. The purpose is to permit people to carry on, to muddle through. So consultation is easy.

But not always. For many years, one of my jobs in Chelsea was to consult weekly with a child protection program that was under contract with the Department of Social Services, the state agency with the unhappy job of preventing child abuse.

Social workers, young women for the most part, often just out of school, often themselves the children of privilege, with a mix of the arrogance of new credentials, untested idealism (all too ready to peel off, leaving a crust of cynicism), a romanticization about ethnic minorities, and naked racism, these fresh professionals are forced to act like cops. With their own all-too-current ambivalence about their own parents and commanding powers they never dreamed they could have, it is often they who decide when to rupture the delicate web, rendered sacred by the boilerplated millennia of biological law, between a mother and her child.

Of course they have supervisors, and there is a burdensome array of courtroom activity around such a decision, and they occasionally have consultants.

Is it ever necessary to remove a child from a home? Of course. Children are often at risk. They have been raped, brutalized, exploited, dropped from windows, left in back alleys—sometimes by their own mothers. Is the decision to take a child a precise reflection of that risk? No, it cannot be. The decisions are always subjective, arbitrary, swept up by bureaucratic momentum and, when looked at systematically, capricious.

At the heart of much of the problem of protective work lies a basic confusion, a conceptual contradiction that is pervasive and invisible. It has to do with the nature of error. Psychiatric social work remains in the shadow of psychiatry. Its formulations generally rely on the language and grammar established by the psychiatric temple guards of psychotherapy. And psychotherapy is the house tool, not casework or community organizing. Therapy, treatment for a disorder, correction of pathology, particularly if paid for by insurance or Medicaid, require a *diagnosis*: a specific and exclusive condition defined by medical practitioners. Historically, politically, functionally, and conceptually, social work emerges from a medical model and remains beholden to it.

The most egregious mistake in the medical tradition is called by philosophers *Type II.* This type of error involves the exclusion of a hypothesis that happens to be true, as compared to *Type I* errors, which involve the acceptance of a hypothesis that turns out to be false. Malpractice experience demonstrates that it is better to order a thousand unnecessary procedures, including hazardous ones, than to miss a single case of cancer. The false positive does not haunt hospitals as much as the false negative. Doctors and social workers in their sphere run less of a risk when they see more pathology than less.

Never mind, for the moment, the iatrogenic outrages committed in the name of Type II; it is central to the culture of medicine. The legal tradition, on the other hand, is dominated by a preoccupation with avoiding Type I errors. The most sacred tenet of Anglo-Saxon law is the presumption of innocence: "It is better that a thousand guilty men go free than one innocent man hang."

The essential problem with child protective work is that it wears a Type II mantle in dealing with a Type I phenomenon. The abuse of a child is a crime and, increasingly, the consequence of identifying a situation of abuse involves not only the placement of a child in foster care but the prosecution of the parent as well. In some states, it is mandatory to notify the district attorney of any circumstance of substantiated abuse.

Protective workers live in terror that a protective case that they have not "substantiated" will wind up with a brutalized or dead child. They do *not* live in the same terror that the state took a child from a mother unnecessarily. Either way, however, it is these underpaid, overworked, and overwhelmed workers who bear the responsibility and take the blame.

The judicial proceedings around "care and protection petitions," which result in the formal removal of the child from an abusive parent, serve only to concretize judgments and lock them in place. The record keeping, the notes, the very thoughts of the social worker investigating a situation of suspected abuse are predicated on the possibility of an eventual subpoena. They never reflect confusion or ambiguity. A case becomes a brief, and the first inclination becomes rigid with supporting facts.

As a consultant, I did not have the authority to explore the back alleys of a worker's psychosocial history, but I sometimes did so nevertheless. More often, I merely suspected they were dark and complex through such hints as an inordinate amount of anger or contempt being expressed about, for example, a mother being too depressed to praise a child's drawing.

I rarely indulged the instinct to say, "Tell me about *your* mother's depression." Safer and possibly more effective was to get more details about the case mother, so she would not remain so ambiguously outlined as to invite projection of the worker's own issues. Instead of remaining at the abstract, blank-screen level of "a depressed mother," the case might focus on that particular depressed mother. I would also wonder (as if to suggest that the worker him- or herself be curious about it as well) *why* the mother was depressed. This process does not always work and is not even available to most protective workers, so that once they or their supervisors make such judgments, the door has been left open for vast numbers of low-income mothers to be thought of as "bad" because so many middle-class professionals have never forgiven their own mothers for . . . whatever.

One learns to read between the lines of psychological jargon to see whether the client is liked or not. The vocabulary of mother-hating is endless. She can be an "icebox mother" or a "smothering" one, or "ambivalent," or, the most damned of all, "borderline." She may be psychotic, but if she is seen as motivated, i.e., not surly to the worker, she is likely to be liked. If she cancels appointments, or just doesn't show up, or worse, is not at home when the worker makes a home visit, she is seen as *not motivated.* This is particularly damning if the worker must report a certain level of "productivity," i.e., direct client contacts, to meet a quota and justify his or her salary.

If the worker is openly despised or called names, the client is very likely not to be liked. I have seen situations of overt abuse in which the child remained with a parent who was "motivated and cooperative" (i.e., liked). And I have seen situations in which a child who was in no danger but was "overindulged" was placed in foster care because the mother refused to accept therapy. In another case, a child was removed from his mother because she had the "poor judgment" to move from one apartment that had lead paint on the walls to another that was *subsequently* discovered to be coated with lead-based paint.

The tools and powers of professionalism are endless. There is a phenomenon that vastly enhances and simplifies the terrible power of protective work, the "voluntary" placement. A parent is told that she can voluntarily place the child who is thought to be at risk and thus avoid going to court. It is actually the worker who would prefer to avoid going to court, a time-consuming process involving much preparation and the risks of cross-examination by a lawyer, generally court-appointed to the parent but, at times, aggressive.

The mother is often not told that once placed voluntarily, i.e., ostensibly at her initiative, the child may not just as voluntarily be returned home. In Massachusetts, once a child is in the jurisdiction of the Department of Social Services, it remains the agency's prerogative to keep or return the child.

As soon as the child is voluntarily placed, welfare payments cease. This often comes as a surprise to the mother. In a not-unusual case, a mother in Chelsea whose children were placed in foster care could no longer afford the apartment she had while receiving AFDC and had to move to a smaller one. Because the smaller apartment was considered inappropriate for a child, the placement became permanent on the basis of the mother's inability to provide adequate housing.

Every protective service worker has his or her own horror story about foster placements. Children are often placed in one foster family after another and abused in one family after another. Whatever neglect or abuse may have taken place in the child's family of origin has become so confounded by subsequent developments that a disturbed adult has been ordained by the very apparatus designed to prevent one from emerging.

And yet, and yet, children must be protected. Every society deserving to be called humane has some means for saying, "This must not happen," when a child is in danger. In this alienated, fragmented, racist, over-bureaucratized, over-professionalized sliver of human space and time, social workers have been delegated this most difficult and disagreeable work.

This society prefers to ignore such contradictions. It generates the poverty that creates abuse and neglect and then blames the victim, who in the end blames her- or himself. And this rigid, jagged societal violence is thinly coated with a patina of professionalism.

Just as the health or sickness of a society can be best gauged by the health or sickness of its mothers, so can its misery. Motherhood is the isthmus of human time, where the quality, the purpose, the essence of our existence are finely etched.

I would say "parenthood" if I could, if androgyny had come to rock the cradle. But it has not. Even in those families in which men utter the words of gender equity and claim an equal share of the burdens of parenting, too often their actual behavior differs little from that of men who disdain it.

If a sane society treats the raising of its children as its most important purpose, then it must treat its mothers as its most cherished members. This is what Babel meant by the "palace of motherhood"; they should be our royalty.

This is not the case in Chelsea. To be a mother in Chelsea is to be swept along a rocky current holding an egg aloft. People on the shore look the other way.

I think about Queenie a lot.

I had been in Chelsea only a couple of years when a letter came from a probation officer in another state. A 37-year-old woman was being transferred to the jurisdiction of the Chelsea District Court with an order for mandatory treatment at the local mental health agency. She had been found not guilty by reason of insanity for the shooting death of her seven-year-old son eight months earlier. She was being released from the state hospital to return "home" at her request. She was now my patient.

A letter from the state hospital followed, and within a few weeks, Queenie was sitting opposite me in the clinic. She was thin and pale. Her naturally blond hair was cut short. She wore no lipstick, but her eyebrows were thinly penciled over blue eyes that narrowed frequently. Her thin lips were set against her teeth, so that lines of tension were lightly drawn around her mouth. She wore tight stretch jeans and a sweater. At one time, she must have been very beautiful.

"You know I killed my son." It was half question, half statement.

"Yes."

"What else do you want to know?"

"I want to know who you are. And I suppose I want to know how it happened."

"I can't tell you. Because I don't remember. They gave me a lot of shock treatments. But I know I shot him. I must have shot him. And then I shot myself, here in the chest. But I didn't die. They patched me up and sent me to the state hospital. I kept trying to die. I tried to hang myself. I tried to choke on a pillowcase. I tried banging my head against the wall. They kept me tied down when they couldn't watch me day and night, and then they gave me shock after shock until I stopped trying to kill myself."

"Do you want to die now?"

"I always want to die. But I finally decided that God didn't want me to. But if you send me back to the hospital, I would find a way to kill myself."

"If I thought you were going to kill yourself, I would have to send you to the hospital. I can't let you die."

"That's what everybody said over and over again. 'We can't let you die.' I let my son die. I killed him. If you want me to talk to you, if you want to be my doctor, you have to promise not to send me to the hospital."

I paused a long time. It was not entirely rational and certainly not a responsible thing to do, but I finally said, "I promise."

She was a Chelsea child, born of alcoholics, raped by her brother, raped by her father, and finally rejected by her mother when she was a teenager. She had a succession of lovers, a succession of husbands, and a succession of children, Terry being the youngest. The two oldest were placed in foster care as toddlers because of her alcoholism. She had a long history of drinking and depression, and when raped by her father at age 14, she had tried to kill herself by cutting her wrists.

The last of the men in her life was Terry's father. He took her to the Southwest, where he was able to find work. For a half dozen years, they had a secure and stable life, and Queenie did not drink. It was a whole new existence for her. She enjoyed being a housewife and mother, and Terry seemed to be a bright and happy little boy. Chelsea was a million miles away. She dared to hope that she herself could be happy.

She described it all as if it were scratched in sand with a thumbnail. There are millions of volumes of emotion at every turn of a life. Shakespeare, Proust, James, Rembrandt, Mozart, and other artists would stop at every detail of such a story and let it burst into life. But there were so many details, and the emotions around each one were so complex and painful, that she must have used reservoirs of energy to keep her story at that level of adumbration—an outline, flat and superficial.

I did not want to ask Queenie to tell me how it felt when her children were placed or when she was raped by her father or her brother or thrown out by her mother or seduced and abandoned by one man after another. I could not ask for the emotional coloring around each of those events any more than I could ask, "What is it like to kill your son?" If you are going to act as one of God's spies in the lives of the oppressed, you must be very, very patient. Emotions glint through murky layers like a lost doubloon in a sunken shipwreck. They cannot be plucked or plundered, and they sometimes disappear when looked at too directly.

Tears are too gross a signal of emotion, and a woman like Queenie works hard to keep her eyes dry. She said once, "I'm afraid if I start to cry I would never stop." One has to seek for emotion in a face like hers as if watching a slow-motion film that has been speeded up to real time. The eye sees and the mind recalls fleeting details that an act of mental will is required to remember.

When Queenie spoke of "hope," the camera saw a look of so much pain and misery pass over her face so quickly that one would need to have known that hope was the worst of all the torments in Pandora's box to have seen it at all.

Eventually, Terry's father left Queenie and their son, as perhaps she always knew he would. But she was not crushed. She did not start drinking. She got herself on welfare, kept her cottage, and continued to care for her son, who, though heartbroken that his father had left, was sufficiently attached to Queenie that he too did not let the abandonment shatter the texture of a secure life. They were not, after all, the only impoverished mother and child in the world. They carried on. One more lost man in her life was not a tragedy, and she had her son.

What she remembers of *that* morning was that Terry left to wait for the school bus down the street. A few minutes later, he returned. He was weeping, "crying very hard," she said, so hard that it was almost impossible to find out what happened. All she could remember was that there had been some altercation with his friends at the bus stop. It was probably one of those fleeting heartbreaks in the lives of children, forgotten minutes later, but at the time feeling like the end of the world. Ordinarily, a parent would have found some way to permit the moment to pass. A smile, a hug, a "there, there," maybe a cookie, or even no response at all would have been fine.

At worst, another rejection—"Don't bother me; go to school"— would have been *good enough*. But some massive switch was thrown in Queenie's mind at the sight of her son wracked with tears. Maybe she saw him and herself suddenly set against the jagged trail of a lifetime of misery. Maybe the *dailyness* of her life, its stolid *busyness* that permitted her to carry on without sentience to all she had suffered, was jarred into stillness. Maybe there was a sudden perception of the endless pain she was yet to suffer, the endless pain her son might yet suffer, the endless pain in life itself.

She does not remember what she thought or felt, only that she began to weep uncontrollably herself. And that's all she remembered for a long time. But she knows her son was dead and that she shot herself. She remembers trying to kill herself in jail and throughout a succession of locked hospital units. And she remembers endless sessions of court hearings that she did not pay attention to or understand or care about. She remembers being taken to one electroconvulsive treatment after another, until months went by in searing confusion. And now she was back in Chelsea where it all began.

After a while, I began to believe, as she did, that her life was consigned to blight. Her own law, "Queenie's Law," was that if anything bad could happen to anyone, it would happen to her. She got a job at one of the more prestigious factories in Chelsea. Her pay was good for factory work, but the working conditions were terrible. It was always 90 degrees or more in the plant, and the noise and confusion were infernal. Stepping back from a work table one day, she fell down several steps through an open hatch in the floor. She injured her back and was in chronic pain for years afterward. She was on workers' compensation for a while, and then the company fired her. There was no union, and a suit started by a local attorney went nowhere.

She was walking down a residential street one day a few years later when a dog suddenly rushed out of an alley and without provocation or warning, took a bite out of her thigh. (I have never known domestic dogs as vicious as the ones in Chelsea! Perhaps they are trained that way as watchdogs, or perhaps responding to a sense of invaded territoriality in this dense, tense city, the dogs chained in the front yards always seem ready to leap at one's throat.)

Sitting at her window, which overlooked a busy street corner, she watched as a child running across the street was hit by a speeding car. Her screams blended in with the sounds of screeching brakes. Several months later, again at the window, as if forced to dream the same nightmare, as if the image of a damaged child were forever to be imprinted on the windows of her mind, she saw another child hit by a car, this time to be killed.

As she was lying in her bed one night during a storm watching television, the ceiling above her suddenly collapsed and drenching rains came pouring through. She had just bought the bed on credit with an expensive mattress for her back, and now it was soaked with water, and decades of old plaster and paint were everywhere.

Standing in the street one day, she overheard an alcoholic neighbor with a grudge against a tenant arrange with a drug-addicted teenager to set fire to an apartment. She went to the police, who ignored her. The house was later gutted with flames. The police came to her, insisting that she be a witness. Arrests were made. Later, she received death threats anonymously on the phone and on notes slipped under her door, warning her not to testify.

Her first son, now living in Chelsea, unemployed and alcoholic, found her in a barroom. There was an emotional greeting. Then he turned his back on her and wanted nothing more to do with her.

Her daughter found her and became a neighbor. She was living with an alcoholic, abusive man. She had a child who was temperamental, irritable, and ran from Queenie when she was presented as "Grandma." This did not prevent her daughter from frequently leaving the boy in her charge with no notice. Queenie felt put upon and resentful, but could not bring herself to say so for fear of alienating her daughter.

Other family appeared in her life in Chelsea. A brother, alcoholic and chronically depressed, was often hospitalized for hepatic coma from advanced cirrhosis or after his frequent serious suicide attempts.

A former husband found her in a bar and shouted to the crowd, "Hey, everybody. Here's a fucking broad who killed her son." She ran out into a winter night, leaving her coat behind.

She was befriended by an uncle and aunt. He was bedridden with severe heart disease. Queenie went to the house on a daily basis to nurse him and cook for the couple. They were warm and appreciative until their daughter visited from a distant city and told her to get out, thinking perhaps that she was trying to ingratiate herself into a legacy. Queenie continued to care for them until one day her aunt and uncle announced that she was no longer welcome. When her uncle died, she was not invited to the funeral; she was not mentioned in his will.

And there were men. At times she felt "in love," and once or twice there was talk of marriage. In every case, they turned out to be already married, alcoholic, or abusive. Generally they left her. On one occasion, an ex-convict who had killed a man refused to leave after beating her and threatened to kill her if she tried to get a restraining order.

These were the events of her life in Chelsea and the substance of our "therapy." Life was one crisis after another, often punctuated by a return to drinking. My role was to listen, urge her to stop drinking, rarely and reluctantly give her a few Valium tablets for sleep, tentatively ask if she were suicidal, and remain available for her calls.

In spite of this endless adversity, not only did she manage somehow to survive each blow and pick herself up for the next one, but in each case where it was possible, with her teeth grinding in determination, she fought back.

After the two children were hit by cars on the street before her eyes, she organized an effort to get a stoplight put on the corner. She wrote letters to the newspaper and appeared at hearings in City Hall with petitions on which she had collected a large number of signatures.

Despite the threats and despite a viciously aggressive cross-examination that went on for days at a time, she persisted as a material witness in the arson case. The arsonist was eventually sent to prison.

She went to a neighborhood legal services attorney about the collapse of her ceiling. Despite eviction threats, she held her rent in escrow until the repairs were made.

She got the restraining order against the threatening murderer who was her jealous lover.

But the forces set against the poor do not relent easily. The stoplight was never put up. While the arsonist was imprisoned, the landlord whom she overheard arrange for the fire remained free. She was not evicted, but her rent was raised and she had to find another apartment. Vaguely terrifying calls would come throughout the night. She paid for an unlisted number. Soon the calls came again. Eventually they stopped.

At times, I would see her or talk to her on the phone every day. At other times, weeks and even months would go by without a word. Her daughter, whose son was seen at the clinic, would occasionally tell me that Queenie was drinking again and ask me to call her. She always came in when I asked her to. Sometimes she would ask for pills, Valium or Prozac. I generally gave her what she asked for, but only a few at a time.

I was often worried about her, wondering if she were still alive or if yet another blow from her fearful life had been the ultimate one. She survived, and I watched the lines in her face grow deeper and longer with survival.

But once, only once, in the 15 years I knew her did we both feel that she had come to the absolute edge. It was late on a Friday afternoon, a time, I confess, when I begin to lose interest. The receptionist who took the call knew Queenie's voice, and after years of experience, knew whether a situation was critical. This time she interrupted me in a session and said that Queenie sounded "in trouble."

I was about to say, "Queenie is always in trouble," but something in her tone of voice told me to take the interruption seriously.

"I have to see you," Queenie said. Her speech was slurred. "I've been drinking. I'm sorry. But I have to see you."

She arrived 15 minutes later. Her face looked like the Greek *persona* of tragedy, the visual manifestation of a groan. She rocked back and forth in the chair, wringing her hands. (I suddenly realized why the anguished wring their hands. They are looking for the sensation of their hands being held. They are *holding their own hands.*) I did not ask what happened. I waited.

"It was just a dream. I heard Terry saying over and over again, 'Mommy, stop.' He must have been saying that when I was shooting him. I woke up screaming. I didn't know what to do. I couldn't call you in the middle of the night. There was a half bottle of vodka. Don't be mad at me. I drank it down. I had two blue Valiums left. I took them and passed out. I woke up an hour ago. I forgot the dream at first. I dragged myself out of bed. I knew something terrible had happened, but I didn't know what it was. When I washed my face in the bathroom, I remembered. 'Mommy, stop. Mommy, stop.' And now I can't stop hearing it. You have to put me in the hospital. I don't think I can go on."

She moaned and rocked and wrung her hands. Her face was wet with tears, but she did not sob. As a child, she had learned to cry silently.

I suppose if I had been a woman, I would not have hesitated to put an arm around her and rock with her. Maybe it would have been a good thing to do and maybe not. I do not think it would have been a good thing for *me* to do, as much as every instinct of humanity seemed to call for it. Too many men in the life of this woman and in the lives of every woman have slipped and sidled from the humanity of consolation to the more familiar one of male intimacy, our blind-alley trap.

So I sat and waited, wondering what I should do, what I should say as I heard through the door the restless sounds of a clinic wanting to go home for the weekend.

"She wants to go to the hospital," I said to myself. "*Send her.*" I did not listen. I often do not listen to what I tell myself. I know that sensible caring voice within. I use it on my children, on my patients. "Do the easy thing. Don't take risks. And who do you think you are, anyway?" It is the last note, the challenge to my narcissism, that usually carries the day.

But not today.

I said, "So many times you have told me that if you went back to the hospital, it would be forever. It would be like dying. I know that it would not be forever and that you would be out soon again. But the way you think about it makes me feel that if you went back, something would be lost in you again. We knew this was going to happen someday, that someday the moments of Terry's death, the feelings, would come back and you would have to decide whether you could handle them or not. All those shock treatments were given to you by people who were convinced that you could not stand the memories. But they are yours. You can't walk through life carrying a locked box you're afraid to open. You killed him because you did not want him to have a life of pain, like yours. You killed him because you loved him."

Should I have said that? Sometimes I think it doesn't matter what one says, that what matters at certain moments is the music of the voice. There are tones and rhythms which speak to that other brain with its nose pressed to the window of color, smell, and emotion, translating them into *words*, a foreign currency.

She stopped rocking after a while and said very quietly, "Thank you."

EIGHT

Everyone in medicine likes a classic case, a patient who cuts through the dross of biological variability and presents a textbook picture of "a disease." This assures us of comforting categories with neat boundaries, as opposed to the nebulous states of *dis-ease*, generalities whose manifestations are diffuse if not arbitrary.

Pure types of phenomena are rare. Natural boundaries around everything from ideas to cells are as capricious as those of nations, which open and close in response to signals never entirely understood by migrants and refugees.

Psychiatry, despite the pretenses of a diagnostic system organized to the hundredth of a decimal place, deals after all with human behavior, with all its ideological, cultural, and linguistic ambiguity about what is crazy and what is not. So there was something reassuring about seeing a classic case of what we used to call "involutional melancholia," a mid-life sinkhole draining away one's energy.

At 44, Lorraine had suddenly begun to be obsessed with the size of her mouth. She believed it was growing and her face was becoming distorted with its consuming presence.

Her mouth was entirely normal. This was a somatic delusion, a grotesquely distorted idea about her ordinary body. She would wake up at three or four in the morning, tossing and turning to the obsessional whiplashes of guilt with their fillips of shame. She had no appetite for food and lost weight. She took pleasure in nothing. Her usual pattern of meticulous homemaking was disrupted; dishes lay unwashed in the sink, dust balls rolled under the bed like tumbleweed in a ghost town, and her familiar bathrobe, all that she ever wore now, was beginning to look stained.

When I asked her about suicide, she merely shrugged as if to say, "Of course, but I don't have the energy."

I turned to the imaginary gaggle of adoring students who occasionally dog my steps and, after listing the diagnostic features of the classic case, asked the one who was fidgeting what the treatment should be. Before he could respond, the pushy one with the mouth and myopia asked in a way more aggressive than seemly why the patient was not hospitalized.

One could certainly justify an inpatient admission, I answered defensively. But this was her first episode and we could expect a rapid response to antidepressants. Also, she had a close and supportive family, and psychiatric hospitalization itself can be an emotional trauma as well as financially costly. And don't interrupt.

I prescribed one of the old war-horses of antidepressant medication, a tricyclic, as they are called, as if war-horses pranced around in three-ring circuses. Classic cases should respond in classic ways to classic treatments. I exuded confidence. Family members were beside themselves with gratitude. The patient herself did not care, perhaps did not believe, had given up hope.

I assured her and myself that within six weeks she would be feeling better. Six weeks is a long time, but this form of tricyclic-speed, even with the adjuvant of my mishmash variety of psychotherapy, works slowly. And besides, acute depressions often go away by themselves. We often give ourselves the credit for a good outcome of the natural course of a self-limiting condition.

Lorraine did not improve. Two months went by with the same grinding misery. I use conservative doses of medicine, so I had the leeway of increasing to a level more acceptable to the zealots of pharmacology. There was still no change. I changed horses midstream, switching to a different tricyclic. These closely related drugs represent an arbitrary variation of the juggled molecules, allowing a different company to patent and market a treatment for depression, giving the illusion of choice, the American way in medicine as well as soap and politics. Sometimes switching medications works. But with Lorraine, there was still no improvement.

The question of suicide was becoming more central. Lorraine had gone from wishes that she not wake up in the morning, the morning that crept like a killer around the edges of shades at dawn, to more specific thoughts about swallowing large numbers of pills. The imaginary student was no longer around, so I could suggest hospitalization without too much loss of face. Her husband was agreeable. He was a postal worker with insurance and had heard from a friend whose wife had had the "same" condition that there was a good private hospital up the river. It would not have been my first choice. I would have preferred one of the small units of general hospitals overrun with students and nurses and the verisimilitude of acute medical care. The alternatives in private care are the asylums now housed in the former mansions of the owners of the rum-running, slave-peddling, opium-dealing clipper ships that made Boston great.

The place he had selected was notorious for its use of ECT, or electric shock treatment, the quickest and most profitable treatment for an emotional life gone awry. The Department of Mental Health had made an abortive effort to pull their license when they were found to be treating a 14-year-old boy with shock treatments for his marijuana habit. The hospital's lawyers were apparently better than the state's; they successfully argued that there can be an underlying depression with marijuana abuse and that ECT is an appropriate treatment for depression.

We like to say "electro-convulsive treatment" to avoid the more shocking and less palatable name. In fact, with the use of curare-like drugs (also used to poison darts in the Amazon) and general anesthesia (used in another and more perilous habitat), there are no convulsions, only the barest flick upward of the great toes to indicate that the brain has indeed been shocked.

It can be, despite its lack of elegance and its risks, an appropriate treatment for depression, if by appropriate one means the kick to a sluggish starter that sometimes gets it going again. Depressed people begin to wear out those around them as well as themselves, and with "compassion fatigue," the temptation to shake them out of their misery becomes very strong. When psychiatrists do the shaking, they use ECT.

In fact, the patients for whom it is most useful and least destructive are those like Lorraine, acute-onset, agitated, and depressed people with somatic delusions who do not respond to medication. Rather than argue with her husband about "shock mills," and since he felt strongly about this "nice" place, which reportedly served gourmet meals, I arranged for her admission and expected that my therapeutic failure would be their triumph.

Several weeks later, she was discharged back to my care. This time *I* was shocked. I expected to see a symptom-free enthusiast for ECT. I found a woman who, despite a dozen and a half treatments, was still depressed and still deluded. She was a little confused at first and less articulate about her complaints, but essentially the same. And when the confusion completely cleared, she was entirely the same.

While I had the comforting assurance that ECT's therapeutic impotence was as great as mine, I was left with a very unhappy patient who would not get better. The imaginary gaggle of students was long gone, so I elected to offer her some sedation at least, with Valium. She reported she felt "better" and was able to sleep, but remained deluded and depressed.

We continued to meet on a regular basis and one day were focusing on her anger. She was angry with her husband for a number of reasons to which she had alluded in the past: a few affairs, some drinking, his demandingness, and now added to the litany, his sloppiness. Did sloppiness, I asked, adjusting my tie, belong with affairs and drinking? He was always starting household tasks, she said, and leaving them half finished, the worst being the business with the walls.

"What business with the walls?" I asked to be polite.

"For months he's been coming home after work and spending about ten minutes before supper blowtorching the walls and scraping the paint off. He leaves the mess for me to clean up, and the stink is terrible."

I experienced a sudden sensation in my stomach. It is called "sinking" in books, but feels more like nausea. After a moment, I asked, "Why is he doing that?"

"Because they told us when we moved in that there was lead paint on the walls and we had to get it off."

In medical school, we were taught only a few bare facts about lead. It was not a matter of great interest to our professors, who were researching esoteric metabolic disorders. We were told to look for a blue edging to the gums and X-ray densities in the long bones of children who had developed acute encephalopathy. We were not taught about the huge numbers of children whose marginal elevations in lead levels affected their learning and behavior. And we were not told about the effects of lead on the emotional lives of adults. But I knew that lead affected the nervous system as well as the kidneys, and I vaguely knew that the very worst way to deal with lead paint on the walls of a house is to blister it with a blowtorch and scrape it off, creating a virtual aerosol of lead fumes and dust.

"Lorraine, I think I know why you have been suffering so much. You may be lead poisoned."

She thought that was interesting, but she suggested that I speak to her husband.

I don't know why just because one changes the focus from therapy to public health, one has to give up all one's finely tuned communication and family dynamics skills. I called her husband at work and said, "Listen, you're poisoning your wife."

He responded, perhaps predictably, "You listen to me, you fucking quack. I know how to take old paint off. Don't blame me for Lorraine's sickness. You've been jerking her around for six months with your fucking pills, and now you're making her a Valium addict. You haven't done a thing for her." And he hung up.

Lorraine was listening to this interchange with the closest thing to amusement I had ever seen on her face.

When I called her husband back at home, I was more rational and calmly explained that there might be a little more lead in the air than was good for everybody and suggested we check the kids as well as Lorraine, and maybe even him. He apologized for calling me a "fucking quack." (I am always wary of apologies that carry a repetition of the insult.) In a few days, we had checked the family's lead levels. Lorraine, being in the house all day and cleaning up the old paint while breathing in the dust, had an elevated blood lead level. Her husband and the kids were "in the normal range."

Now I had to think. Here appeared to be a textbook case of involutional melancholia, complete with the appropriate intrapsychic and family dynamics, including the emergence of instinctual rage internalized as depression after the breakdown of obsessional defenses, and all the time she was lead poisoned.

I thought, if this "classic" case was largely, if not primarily, a result of lead poisoning, what about everybody else who came to the clinic, the *non*-classic cases? How much lead was in the bodies of all the other depressed and anxious people, all the hyperactive kids and acting-out adolescents, the psychotic adults and the demented elderly?

I began taking blood samples from everybody who came to the clinic. At times it seemed like Transylvania Station. The state Department of Public Health's laboratory tested blood free for anyone under the age of 12 and provided plastic pipettes, finger puncture equipment, and even mailing envelopes at no cost. So, for a while, everyone in the clinic was declared to be under 12 years of age.

When the results started to come back, I discovered that these 12-year-olds of all ages—psychotic, borderline, neurotic, panic-stricken, impulse-ridden, demented—almost all had elevated lead levels.

The federal government had decided at that time that a blood lead level of 30 micrograms per 100 cc of blood was toxic; thus a level of 29 was safe. This was before the ground-breaking studies of Herbert Needleman at Children's Hospital in Boston, which determined that there is a straight-line relationship between the amount of lead in the body and careful measures of disturbed behavior and learning problems. There is no such thing as a normal or non-toxic level of lead in the human body; any exposure of a child's nervous system to lead will have some effect. Interestingly, the federally defined "acceptable" level of lead has since been lowered.

Almost all of the readings I obtained from my patients at the clinic were in the 20s. Fortunately, this was not high enough by federal standards to be considered treatable. The treatment, using chelating agents, which combine with the lead in the blood and permit its excretion through the kidneys, is useful only for acute intoxication, not for chronic, ongoing exposure during which the lead accumulates in the bones as well as the kidneys and brain. These chelating agents are themselves toxic to the kidneys, and there have been occasions when their use precipitated acute poisoning of the brain. In a person who has had prolonged exposure to a marginal amount of lead that has gradually accumulated in the bones, the sudden excretion of the lead into the blood can cause a subsequent surge at a level high enough to cause a neurotoxicity that had not been present before.

This is not unlike the acute poisonings that occur when a house is being "deleaded," and the paint that was formerly on the walls suddenly becomes part of the ambient dust. This is what happened to poor Lorraine. The only effective treatment is prevention.

Here I was working at a clinic in Chelsea, running around with my grab bag of drugs and psychotherapy and *kindness*, when I should have been thinking about lead.

Where is the lead in Chelsea found? Where *isn't* the lead in Chelsea found? Ninety percent of the homes in the city have lead paint somewhere on their surfaces. Lead batteries have accumulated in the city's dumps. Lead from batteries and paint accumulates in the dust and soil following one fire after another. The basest of base metals, it never breaks down, which is why it should have been left below the surface of the earth where it belongs rather than being mined by centuries of slaves to line aqueducts, sweeten wine, cast bullets, strengthen paint, and generate electricity for a species of biology *intoxicated* by its own inventiveness and staggering in a drunken lust for profit.

I became an expert in lead. I soon learned that the city had its own unique source. Chelsea bears on its back the Mystic-Tobin Bridge like the true cross. Built in the fifties to speed North Shore commuters to Boston, it spans and splits the city in half. Over time, the bridge was painted and repainted with lead to cut down on the need for more frequent coatings of pigment. But with the seasons and the tintinnabulations of rush-hour traffic over the years, bits of paint would crumble and fall to the already less-than-virginal earth below. The space directly below the bridge was by common consent and tradition a playground and parking area. Contiguous to it are the Williams School, a combined elementary and middle school, a day-care center called the Kangaroo's Pouch, some vegetable gardens, and the back porches of several hundred dwellings—low income, of course.

The soil under the bridge was tested at 3000 parts lead per million parts

of other ingredients. The federal government, no zealot when it comes to the environment, fearing the sin of over-scrupulousness and the ire of the lead industry, had determined that the acceptable level of lead in soil was 500 parts per million. The bridge, the longest in New England, was poisoning the people.

A new mayor in town, a young man of its own soil, agreed to sign a letter to the Massachusetts Port Authority complaining about the bridge as a source of lead toxicity. After a delay of several weeks, the administrator of the Authority wrote back that while they did not accept any responsibility for having exposed the citizens of Chelsea to the danger of lead poisoning, they would stop using lead-based paint and use something safer in the future. In essence, the letter stated that they had done nothing wrong but would stop doing it.

It was a triumph. Reason and virtue had blown their trumpets at the gates of Authority, and Authority had knelt in defeat without even the pretense of conflict.

"That was easy," I said to myself. A spigot of pathology had been turned off with the slightest effort. Even Dr. Snow, the father of public health, had to work harder to break the handle of the Broad Street pump in 1854.

I put away the public health helmet and returned to being a clinician. This included the ongoing care of Lorraine. Her depression improved slightly after her blood lead level dropped to the normally elevated standards of her fellow citizens, but she never actually returned to a normal state of mind. This unhappy fact tended to confirm my suspicion that with adults as well as children, once the delicate filigree of nerves in the brain is impacted by lead, it never fully recovers. Lead poisoning is like being bashed in the head with a baseball bat.

I did what I could for Lorraine, and while I continued to suspect that some part of the grinding misery and explosive impulsivity I ministered to in my other patients was rooted in lead as well, I continued my customary treatments. I imagine that after he broke the handle of the Broad Street pump, Dr. Snow went back to treating his patients with leeches and bloodletting and purgatives or whatever they used then to torment people in the name of medicine.

Certainly, after being a Marxist revolutionary, Rudolf Virchow, the "father of pathology," returned to the morgue where there were at least no worries about the efficacy and safety of his ministrations. Even Dr. Guevara might have given an aspirin or two after the Cuban revolution. So it should surprise no one that after dabbling more or less satisfactorily on the ramparts, I could return to a more or less conventional practice of psychiatry.

Time goes by. The leaves on the calendar are blown away by the high-powered fan behind the movie camera. About a year and a half later, I was driving to work on a summer morning. I used, I confess, the Mystic-Tobin Bridge in the mornings, a fast drive against the rush-hour traffic with a fleeting glimpse of the U.S.S. Constitution and gulls swooping over the dappled waters of Boston Harbor.

Ahead of me was a new sign. Writ large in black on orange were the words "BRIDGE CLEANING AHEAD: CLOSE YOUR WINDOWS." I am a good citizen. I rolled up my car windows. A hundred feet later, I saw a canvas-enclosed cubicle in which workers wearing space suits were using blasting equipment. A plume of black grit rose from the top of the enclosure and fell on the surface of the bridge, onto passing cars and onto the D Street projects in Charlestown below that section of the span.

Every once in a while, in a fleeting fit of automotive vanity, I drive through a car wash. I had done so two days earlier and cast a small curse on the bridge cleaners for scattering their waste on the surface of my four-year-old Chevrolet.

Thirty seconds later, still above the Mystic River, I experienced that old sinking sensation in the stomach. "That's lead," I said aloud.

When I got to the clinic, I called the Massachusetts Port Authority, the "owner" of the bridge. It was like calling the Vatican, or a taste of Kafka. Finally, after being passed through four secretaries who had not yet had their coffee, I was given to the chief engineer of Massport. In response to my inquiry, he said, "This is not my doing. It was planned before I took this job. Apparently, a couple of years ago, there was a fuss in Chelsea about lead paint on the bridge. We decided to switch to a zinc-based paint, but zinc does not adhere to lead, so we have to blast off the old paint down to the bare metal. If there has been any damage to your car, you can apply to the Authority for reimbursement."

I tried to sound calm. "I'm not really concerned about my car, but you are blasting lead paint onto people's houses."

"We've taken precautions to protect the public. The enclosures we use are adapted from the ones used on the Golden Gate Bridge. We went out there to study them."

I responded, "The enclosures aren't working and you know they aren't. You're warning drivers to close their windows. You can see the stuff coming out. The whole idea was to prevent lead poisoning and you're making things worse."

A North Atlantic chill entered the voice of the Authority. "May I ask what concern this is of yours?"

"I'm a doctor. I am going to be treating the people who are poisoned by your bridge cleaning." Notice that I did not say I was a psychiatrist, thereby inviting an irrational response.

"Thank you for your interest, doctor, but we know what we are doing." Click!

I imagined that in just such a way the London water commissioner told Dr. Snow that *they* knew what *they* were doing and to mind his own medical business. And I imagine that he trembled with the same sense of frustrated rage and a fantasy of taking violent action.

There was no pump handle to break to neatly and cleanly stop a cholera epidemic. I did, however, have an image of myself in a black sweater and wool cap crawling along the catwalk of the bridge at midnight with a pound of sugar to pour into the fuel tanks of the blasting generators. But this was only a fleeting fantasy, lasting no more than several entire nights.

I told the story to a journalist friend, who said in his nondirective way, "Here's what you have to do. On no more than one typewritten page, write what lead is, how it affects the body, why you are worried about it, and what is happening on the bridge. Send it to the following people."

One page. Condensing the history of lead poisoning into one page was a challenge, but I did it and sent my elixir of "Massport is poisoning the children of Chelsea with lead" to the five editors suggested by my friend, along with a cover letter mentioning his door-opening name.

None of them called or wrote back, but a secretary in the clinic had a brother who worked at a TV station. She called him, and several hours later somebody from the investigative team at one of the channels called. He was not sure there was a story here, but the legislature was not in session and there was not much else to investigate. He asked a few questions and then suggested taking a shot of me in front of the bridge; this would have required my being suspended by a helicopter above the Mystic River, so we settled for my standing in front of the clinic.

There I was surrounded by a claque of giggling children in front of a camera answering an interviewer's questions about what lead is, how it affects the body, and what my concerns about the bridge were. The next shot was of the chief engineer of Massport. He had shed his chill for the evening news and was smiling behind his desk with the flags of the Commonwealth and the USA behind him. He was calm and reassuring, saying, "We are using state-of-the-art equipment." The last shot was of the space-suited men on the bridge *pushing a broom.*

Since television defines the news, there subsequently appeared several articles, an editorial, and even a cartoon showing a white rabbit making an "Oh, my god," slap-in-the-head gesture on learning that in order to avoid using lead paint, Massport was scraping it off the bridge onto the people below.

Several weeks later, in response to the publicity, a public meeting was organized by Fair Share, a public interest lobbying group. Several dozen citizens showed up at the Methodist church on Broadway in Chelsea to hear a debate between a representative of Massport and myself.

The man from Massport wore a perpetual smile slung between red cheeks over a vested suit. He was the public information officer, the "mouth" of the Authority. He did not want to fight. He introduced himself to me before the meeting and stretching his smile to the limit, said, "I think we should avoid making this adversarial." I smiled back noncommittally.

I was asked to speak first, the prosecution. I was low-keyed and professional, simply describing lead poisoning as the worst public health menace of all time. (I'm not sure that's true, but it was not a time for quibbling.)

The man from Massport seemed to be sweating under his three-piece suit, but he was still smiling. He said when he got to the podium that he did not disagree with anything "the doctor" had said about lead, but Massport had been scrupulous and responsible in protecting the public. "In fact, we have state-of-the-art equipment," etc., etc.

I declined a rebuttal, allowing more time for discussion. There were a few questions about details and then a woman raised her hand. A pale three-year-old girl leaned against her. The woman got up and said in a shaky voice that this was the second summer that her daughter had to have injections of chelating agents for lead poisoning. The house had been checked for lead paint and there was none. They lived on Chestnut Street next to the bridge. She couldn't stand to hear her daughter crying about the injections. The child was tired all the time. At this point, her voice quavered. "I was very upset when I learned that the bridge had lead on it and I think . . . I think that . . . ," and she burst into tears, perhaps not really knowing what she thought.

The room was silent. The man from Massport was not now smiling, but he stood resolutely at the podium. He must have said to himself, "This is what I'm being paid for." Aloud he said: "The Massachusetts Port Authority accepts no responsibility for your child's condition. There is no reason to assume that the lead in your child's body came from the bridge. There are other sources of lead in this community, and a responsible parent can make certain that a child does not ingest lead."

I experienced a flash of a Brooklyn schoolyard instinct to take a swing at him, but it passed immediately. I actually felt sorry for the son of a bitch. I could imagine the briefing with his supervisors, who must have told him what to say if there were the slightest hint of liability in a particular case. It sounded memorized or electronic, and maybe if he were to keep his job, it was the only thing he could have said. But it was wrong.

The audience stirred. Eyes narrowed. No one spoke for about ten seconds. Then a big guy in the back got up. "All right," he said. "You go back and tell your buddies at Massport that if they don't stop what they're doing on the bridge, we're going to go up there and turn those blasters up your ass."

I have no romantic fantasies about the possibilities of class struggle. I have none now and had none then, but when that man sat down and the hall exploded in shouts and applause, I saw in my mind's eye the walls of the Methodist church separating like a painted curtain. I saw Fidel and Nat Turner, Rosa Luxemburg and Joe Hill, Mother Jones and Spartacus; I saw thousands of poor people marching up the Third Street ramp, stopping traffic in all directions, and the bridge trembling to the rhythm of their feet, with police cars helpless and helicopters hovering, their pilots screaming to anchormen that the bridge had been taken by the people. How quick these dreams are, no more than a skipped heart beat.

But reality moves at a more ponderous pace, its haunches barely seen to shift. The mayor was asked to convene a committee of Chelsea citizens to "work with" the planners of Massport to come to a resolution. Blasting was suspended until agreement could be reached. I became an honorary citizen of Chelsea for this purpose and, as "the doctor," was given the job of coming up with the demands the committee should make.

We held lots of meetings in the evening, and I confess that my biggest problem with them was not the late hours and the endless talk and the homework but the goddamned cigarette smoke. At one meeting, I almost exploded to the people in the room that we were dealing with issues of health and pollution, and therefore . . . but I didn't want to scare them off.

Eventually, we came up with a list of conditions, including constant air monitoring for lead, house-to-house checks of families near the bridge, and the redesign of the fancy San Francisco enclosures. Massport more or less adhered to these conditions, but it turned out that some of the bridge's oblique spans could not be enclosed and therefore had to be repainted with lead paint after all.

The dust of Chelsea continues to be full of lead and children continue to be poisoned. Prevention in a devastated environment is an endless struggle with a hydra-headed beast, only some of whose heads are human. To me, the struggle is embodied in a simple, straightforward premise: *We cannot trust the institutions around us.* Massport was more interested in moving cars across the bridge than preventing the destruction of children. The agency that was supposed to oversee the health effects of Massport's activities was the Department of Environmental Quality Engineering (now called the Department of Environmental Protection). They never appeared interested or concerned during the entire process. Shortly after these events, the smiling man from Massport was given an important job in that "watchdog" agency.

I learned about lead the way a child learns about sex. The revelation was not that it existed, but that *there was so much of it.* It reminded me of the scene in Heller's *Catch 22* in which Yossarian comes upon an injured airman. He carefully bandages the boy's bleeding leg, saying, "There, there," to his murmuring. He hears the boy say that he is cold and is about to adjust a flight jacket over him when the boy's guts suddenly spill out. Yossarian, trying to hold them in place, can only repeat, "There, there. There, there."

When I began to realize how vast and vastly destructive the problem of lead was in Chelsea, I had a sense of a curtain being pulled back on a scene of devastation, in one small corner of which I was performing a job that seemed as irrelevant as Yossarian's bandaging the leg wound.

Lead, I later learned, was not Chelsea's only environmental problem.

Ramón was known to everyone in Chelsea. You could hear him shouting to himself a block away over the noise of the Broadway traffic. His speech, both in Spanish and English, had an abrupt, machine gun-like staccato pattern with a dactylic prosody. He made what the psychopathologists call "clang associations." One had to be impressed with the endless, senseless ingenuity with which words poured out of him. It was as if some part of his nervous system had been dammed up with language and now, like a flooded stream, was rushing wildly past, while memory, perception, experience, and thought itself stood by stunned on its banks.

He would occasionally giggle, perhaps at the playfulness of his own verbiage, but one would never know. He was incapable of carrying on a conversation and if, rarely, he would respond to a question with an apt word or two, it was immediately followed by another burst of meaningless verbal ordinance.

He was, of course, called "schizophrenic" and had been repeatedly hospitalized in Boston as well as in New York and Puerto Rico. It was said that he once killed a man, and people were frightened of him. But on one occasion when I saw him with his family, his three-year-old niece, indifferent to his psychotic patter, climbed on his knees and cuddled on his lap, as if she had done it hundreds of times before with no one being concerned for her safety.

His psychopharmacological treatment was a crash course in modern psychiatry, with one tranquilizer or anticonvulsant or mood stabilizer after another thrown at him in different combinations and dosages. Its jumble began to make as much sense as his own verbal behavior.

There was a hypnotic quality to the seamless, scudding, three-beat measures of his speech; if I listened to him for any duration of time, I had to be careful not to fall asleep.

I often tried to find something in the salad of his speech to hang on to, to comment on, to try to converse with. It was not easy. Then one day, I heard him say, ". . . *tu estas calor* ."

"*No, Ramón. No tengo calor* [I'm not warm]."

"What?" he asked.

"I said, '*no tengo calor.*' "

"Why you say that?" he asked.

"I thought you said '*tu estas calor.*' " I was beginning to feel a little psychotic myself at this point.

He said, "*No dije eso* [I didn't say that]."

"What *did* you say?"

"I said, 'I like Tester's Glue.' "

"What?"

"Don't tell my mother."

This "schizophrenic" man, like many others, I soon learned, would buy three tubes of Tester's Airplane Glue, squeeze them into a small paper bag, which he would place (as flight attendants tell us to do) securely over the nose and mouth and then breathe rapidly until the volutes of vapor curled through his brain.

Rocco's Spa down the street did a heavy business in Tester's Glue. No model airplane kits were to be found there.

There have been suggestions that the manufacturers of model airplane glue and other domestic sources of toxic organic solvents should add an irritant that would make it difficult for them to be used as intoxicants. Tester's Glue has no such additive. Nor, as I was soon to learn, was the sniffing of glue the major source of organic solvent neurotoxicity.

Among the employers who thrive on Chelsea's cheap labor and proximity to the gasoline tank farms on its shores are the American Finish and Chemical Company and the Marson Corporation, both of which use volatile organic solvents, such as toluene, benzene, and acetone. The use of these chemicals has to be seen within a broader context.

According to the National Institute of Occupational Safety and Health (NIOSH), nearly ten million workers are exposed to the 49 million tons of industrial solvents produced each year in the U.S. NIOSH describes three levels of chronic toxicity with these products. Type I, of "minimal" severity, involves the subjective experience of fatigue, irritability, memory problems, poor concentration, and mood disturbances. Type II, of "moderate" severity, is manifested by objective personality changes, including loss of impulse control, severe mood abnormalities, and intellectual deficiencies. Finally, the most severe and chronic exposure, Type III, causes dementia. At each level of exposure and before a medical problem emerges, the manifestations of such poisoning are psychiatric.

One of my patients worked in the mixing room of the Marson Corporation. The air was heavy with the sickeningly sweet vapors of substances used to make the quick-setting filler for automobile body repairs. She had constant headaches, could not sleep, reported losing control of her temper with her children, and felt anxious and depressed. (In the fictive world of psychiatric diagnosis, anxiety and depression are separate "disorders." In reality, they are generally found together.) Like many of my patients, she wanted Valium for sleep, which I refused to give her. I thought her working conditions might have had something to do with her distress. She thought so, too, but there was no union and she was afraid to complain.

I found a listing in the phone directory for the regional office of the Occupational Safety and Health Administration (OSHA). The person with whom I spoke informed me that as the worker's physician, I could request the agency's involvement without revealing the identity of the employee if he or she were reluctant to make the complaint.

A day later, I received an easy two-page form on which I noted the patient's symptoms and the name and location of the factory. A week later, I received a copy of a report from OSHA to the management of the Marson Corporation listing 32 separate violations of worker safety and health. The company was given one month to correct the violations; if they were not corrected, penalties would be instituted.

Six weeks later, I was sent a statement from OSHA reporting that their follow-up investigation revealed that most of the violations had been corrected, mainly having to do with venting fans and the use of masks and gloves, but that they would continue to monitor the situation.

This was during the Carter administration and represented the kind of intrusive regulation of the free market that Ronald Reagan's presidency was ordained to repair. I experienced the effects of his repairs a few years later. The American Finish and Chemical Company threatened to fire some workers who were complaining about their exposure to chemicals. The workers had asked for masks and gloves but were told these were not necessary and that they were free to get out and find other work if they couldn't "take it."

A few of the workers, all of whom were Puerto Rican or Central American, decided to call a union, any union. There had been a successful strike shortly before by Local 66 of the Laundry and Dry Cleaning International Union against a mattress manufacturer in town, and there had been a picture in the *Chelsea Record* of the jubilant workers celebrating their pay raise. The unhappy workers at American Finish and Chemical called the same union.

The president of the union later said it was the easiest organizing job he had ever seen. The workers were already organized before the union representative met with them. The company refused to recognize the union or speak with its representative. A strike was called. I was asked to address the workers, about 50 in all, about the health effects of the chemicals to which they were being exposed.

I had been given the list of ingredients and did the research, but standing on a sidewalk, microphone in hand, I found myself not in a scholarly mode. The men already seemed to know that the chemicals were "messing them up." I marched with them and chanted, "WHAT DO WE WANT? A CON-

TRACT! WHEN DO WE WANT IT? NOW!" Truckers driving by honked and raised their fists in support. We cheered in response. When managers drove up to the gate, the police gently parted us as we shouted, "Scab!" at the white-collar workers who were suddenly in the position of having to do the dirty work usually left to Spanish-speaking laborers. The strike was won in a few days. The company was forced to recognize the union and sign a contract that included provisions for the protection of the workers.

I would never have believed during my training to become a psychiatrist that chanting on a sidewalk would be the highest and finest expression of mental health professionalism.

Failure in what I have come to call "psychotoxicology" is much more bitter than success and much easier to come by. By the time there are objective changes in mood, behavior, or intellectual function from organic solvent exposure, the problems are irreversible. As with lead poisoning, the only treatment is prevention.

Carlos's mother walked into the clinic one day and asked to talk to *el doctor*. She knew nothing about intake evaluations or appointments or the differences among social workers, psychologists, and psychiatrists. Anyone who spoke with her would be *el doctor*.

Like a supplicant in a temple, Carlos's mother begged for help. She had heard that the doctors sometimes went to people's houses. Would we, could we, come to see Carlos? I suppose if she had not begged so much, I might have suggested that she try a little harder to bring him to the clinic, that she make an appointment and "do it right." Instead, I apologized to the waiting patients and went to her house on Chestnut Street.

Carlos was 23. His mother had just returned with him from California. His wife had called Carlos's mother in Chelsea to tell her to come and get him out of her house. He was *loco* and she was afraid for her life.

When he had left for California several years earlier to "see the country," he had been fine, better than fine. He had been one of the few Puerto Rican boys to graduate from Chelsea High School. He was smart. He spoke English very well. There was even talk about his going to college, which Carlos's mother, who did not speak English, thought about with a heart swelling with pride and amazement.

But it was not to be. He got a job and, having saved a few hundred dollars, decided to take the bus to California. Once there, he fell in love with a *Chicana*, a Mexican-American woman, and determined to make a life in Los Angeles. They were married, and he got a job in a factory.

Carlos's mother had talked to her daughter-in-law on the phone, but had never met her until this trip of confusion and anxiety and enormous expense. (She was now, for the first time in her life, heavily in debt.)

According to Carlos's mother, he had always been a bright and happy child, a little stubborn at times, but not like the others who used drugs and got into trouble. He had been a "good boy" and now he was like a stranger. He would not talk, just sat and stared all day. He ate and dressed like a machine and then just sat. He would not even watch television. But at times he became frightened for no apparent reason and once ran to the kitchen to get a knife. Now he kept it under his mattress when he slept. When his mother tried to take it from him, he hit her, something he had never done before. Now she was terrified of her own son.

He had no reaction to my coming to the house. He looked at me as if I were on the other side of a pane of glass. I sat next to him on the couch and asked questions quietly in Spanish and English and waited a long time for answers that did not come. After a little while, I arranged for an ambulance and had him taken to the Lindemann Mental Health Center, where he was diagnosed as "catatonic schizophrenic" and given Haldol.

This is not the place to explore the mysteries of psychiatric diagnosis. He certainly looked the way a catatonic schizophrenic is supposed to look. But I remembered a "classic case" at McLean Hospital, who, several days after residents were taken through to see what catatonia looks like, was dead from encephalitis. Even allowing for the blindness of mothers about their sons, it did not seem right that a boy who had been bright and social, who had been able to court and marry a woman from another culture, was now suddenly so absolutely and intractably psychotic. However much Haldol he was given, he did not improve.

Carlos's mother did not know what kind of factory he had worked in, but when I called his wife in California, she told me that it was a place that made "lacquers," and she hated the smell on his breath and, yes, several other men in the factory had "gone mental." And, yes, she would certainly call OSHA or something, and she hung up.

The psychiatry residents at Lindemann were only mildly interested in lacquer. We had entered the age of computer-assisted, two-minute psychiatric diagnoses and polypharmacy. Once thought schizophrenic, a patient would be subjected to a mix of antipsychotic drugs as well as Lithium, anticonvulsants, beta blockers like Inderal, and a little assist from benzodiazepines like Ativan or Klonopin. The preferences are always for the newest drug, the fashions being dictated by the profit margin of the industry. Research grants, continuing education programs, conferences, grand rounds, as well as the "literature" itself, are paid for by pharmaceutical companies who carefully program the attention of psychiatrists to the latest and most profitable drugs.

Nothing worked for Carlos. He was sedated but remained psychotic and was finally discharged back to the community, to his mother, to the clinic, and to a day treatment program. The last was most important because his mother did not have to worry about his sitting around the house or wandering the mean streets of Chelsea while she was at work. Here was one more chronic psychotic citizen of Chelsea, one more blasted mind, one more helpless child-man in the care of one more exhausted mother.

Bringing him to the clinic on a monthly basis to see me was not as much a problem as getting him to go to the day treatment program. Every morning there was a struggle with much cajoling, entreating, and shouting.

And then one morning, about a year and a half after he came home, Carlos's mother lost control and began hitting him with all her strength, all her pent-up fury and frustration and misery. She slapped him again and again. Then he slapped her back so hard that she fell, and he ran from the house moaning.

Again she came to the clinic, tearfully begging for something to be done, for Carlos to be put back in the hospital. But Carlos had run to the bridge that connected Chelsea to East Boston, smaller and more accessible than the Mystic-Tobin Bridge. He ran to the center and jumped into the chilly, lead-colored waters. A picture in the *Boston Herald* showed the State Police diving team trying to rescue him, but Ophelia-like, he eventually submerged and drowned.

I went to the wake a few days later. He looked wonderful in the casket: a handsome, well-dressed, intelligent-looking young man . . . asleep. There were about 50 people in the room. Most of the women were in tears. The men bowed to me as I took a seat in the back. Carlos's mother was kneeling, praying, rocking slightly in front of the casket. A younger woman was next to her. When she saw me, she whispered to Carlos's mother, who immediately whirled to her feet.

"*Doctor*," she wailed. "*Ayudeme* [Help me]!" She ran down the aisle to where I was sitting. I got up. She put her head on my chest and sobbed. I patted her on the back. "*Venga* [Come]," she said. "*Mire* [Look at him]. *No es muerte* [He isn't dead]. Look, he's breathing. Make him wake up. Help him. Help me. Please, doctor. Please talk to him. I beg you."

She tried to drag me down the aisle to the coffin. Several people rushed to her and put their arms around her. A man tried to apologize to me. They took her into the next room, where we could still hear her wailing and sobbing. After a little while, I left.

Long ago, I became accustomed to being at odds with my profession. Being obsessed with poverty as a source of psychopathology does not permit much discourse with psychiatrists who insist that illness is entirely a matter of chemistry. I was tolerated, at times even celebrated, in the condescending way practical men acknowledge issues of social justice. At academic conferences, I played something of the role of the fool at court. I was a lefty, a philosopher, a scholar with a mouth who could be counted on to say something amusing, maybe even incisive or interesting, but never thought to be quite *relevant*. Biological psychiatry had a seriousness, a *correctness* that no social issue, no matter how authoritatively documented, could possibly approach.

Here I now was, stumbling into a whole new dimension of biological psychiatry. I, too, had become interested in chemicals. But try as I could, I was not able to get the serious attention of my colleagues. I wrote an article about neurotoxins and behavior, which reviewed the literature, described some case histories, and offered the modest recommendation that clinicians inquire, as a matter of routine, about the possibility of exposure to neurotoxic substances. Rejected by two psychiatric journals as not being scientific or relevant enough for their readers, it finally appeared in an international journal of medical sociology.

Contemporary psychiatry is not interested in the biochemical abnormalities underlying mental illness unless those abnormalities are inherent and genetic or, as the Nazi psychiatrists used to say, *constitutional*. The economic, social, and political realities that govern our professional life dictate that mental illness not be seen as in any way environmental in origin. And this, I discovered, includes the physical as well as the social environment.

The disinterest on the part of my profession about the effects of chemical pollutants on the nervous system kept pace with that of the government itself.

I was spoiled by my first experience with OSHA during the Carter administration. I pictured something built-in, nonideological, bureaucratized, a permanent apparatus like the fire department or the Library of Congress. But I was wrong, having once again underestimated the power of the Right.

Over the course of a year in 1990, I became aware of a pattern of unusual psychotic episodes. They were only four in number, and I dismissed the first three as probably not psychotoxic events. The fact that three individuals had developed flagrantly psychotic states, with paranoid delusions, auditory hallucinations, and aggressive impulsivity, despite no past history and with seemingly intact prior social lives, had to be called merely "atypical."

But when I saw the fourth such patient who worked in the same place and she, in addition, complained of numbness and tingling in her fingers as well as headaches and blurred vision, I was no longer comfortable. All four made salads at one of the companies that prepared meals for the airlines. The work was hard, with enormous pressures of speed and intrusive supervision, in a setting alternatively stifling and freezing. But the pay was good and, more importantly, the company accepted as Puerto Rican (i.e., American) people who had come from Central America without documents.

The green card is a treasure that many of the Hispanic people of Chelsea do not possess. An employer who does not insist on valid proof of citizenship or a work permit will have no trouble finding workers for any job, no matter how uncomfortable, unsafe, or unhealthy.

But while I understood the plant to be stressful and uncomfortable, I assumed it was, at least, safe and healthy. We were not, after all, talking about lacquers or auto body filler, but arugula salads and *boeuf bourguignonne*. However, when I saw the fourth new patient with an atypical psychosis who worked in the same place, I once again became suspicious. I called OSHA.

I kept a record of my six months of contacts with government agencies around this issue, with dates and names and quotes, but it would be tedious to reproduce and would read too much like satire. We had entered the era of Reagan environmentalism. I will summarize.

First, someone at OSHA told me that the employees themselves had to register a complaint and that I could not do it on their behalf. I protested that I had once done so and understood it was within the regulations. He said he would check and call me back. He never did. When I called back, he did not remember that we had spoken before and had no record of the call. I had by this time told and retold the story dozens of times, so I repeated it once more like a child doing a catechism. With a sigh, the man from OSHA agreed to take the information and see if it deserved an investigation.

"What were they exposed to?"

"I don't know. That's what I want you to find out."

"I'm afraid we can't investigate unless we know what they were exposed to."

"Does that make sense to you?"

"We operate according to official policies and procedures. We don't just go around harassing employers."

"I'm not asking you to harass anyone. I'm asking you to find out what is making my patients sick, and you're telling me that you can't find that out unless you already know."

"We can only intervene with known environmental toxins. Another agency determines whether they are toxic or not."

"What's that?"

"NIOSH, the National Institute of Occupational Safety and Health." "No, I don't have their number."

So I called NIOSH, which was located in Cincinnati. Again, I told the story a dozen times before someone seemed interested. He said, "It certainly sounds like your patients have been exposed to something, but we're not really an enforcement agency. We're a research outfit, and I'm not sure we can get in there."

"Look," I said, "OSHA tells me they can't get in unless you find out what's in there, and you tell me you can't find out what's in there unless they can get in."

"I know it sounds that way. But here's what I'll do. Let me get our mental health expert involved. He can arrange a special investigation. He's a psychiatrist and will be interested in this. He'll call you."

He didn't call, so several weeks later, I called him.

"Oh, yeah. I had a note somewhere about this thing. Let me find it and call you back."

He didn't call, so several weeks later, I called him again.

"Yes, I might be interested in this, but not from the point of view of environmental toxins. I've been collecting instances of what I call 'mass environmental hysteria.' Patients can mimic a whole range of somatizing symptoms, and I find that there are clusters of similar complaints from people who think they are being exposed to toxic chemicals. I would appreciate it if you would send me copies of the records of your four patients."

I said, "I don't have their permission to send copies of their records."

"Oh, you don't need that. Our regulations give us the right to see patients' records without their permission."

"Well, I don't think I want to do that. There may be some immigration problems with some of these people."

"I'm not interested in that."

"I know, but I'm not comfortable sharing their records with a federal agency."

"I can subpoena those records. My regulations give me that right."

I felt a sudden wave of panic. Then I asked, "Tell me something. How are you going to subpoena their records if I don't give you their names?"

There was a long pause. "I have to check with my supervisor. I'll get back to you."

I have had no contact with OSHA or NIOSH ever since and am not likely to. What had once been an apparatus for the protection of workers seems to have become yet another agency for the advancement of neo-fascism.

However, a state agency, the Division of Occupational Hygiene, which did not have the regulatory "muscle" of OSHA, had access to reports about what chemicals could be found on the premises of employers of a certain size. On the basis of my complaint, they shared their report about the chemicals in the food plant with a consultant in environmental health at the Harvard School of Public Health. Six months after I started making official inquiries about the whole thing, a conclusion was reached.

The company, which prepared meals for airlines, was using large amounts of an insecticide containing a substance known as di-thio-carbamate. In the presence of the acidic environment created by the phosphates used in the cleaning of commercial cooking equipment, di-thio-carbamate releases another compound known as carbon disulfide.

The classic textbook of industrial toxicology by Hamilton and Hardy reports on a German study "of no less than fifty patients with carbon disulfide insanity. The early symptoms consisted of headache, dizziness, increasing sense of weariness, loss of strength, transient excitement, and slight delirium very like alcoholic intoxication. Later came deep depression and loss of memory, increasing indifference, and apathy. This might change suddenly to acute mania or delusions of persecution with hallucinations. . . . Some [cases] ended in recovery, others in incurable dementia."

When confronted with this information, the managers of the food preparation plant disclaimed any responsibility for the intoxication of their workers. They insisted that alcohol abuse was more likely the cause. I had no reason to suspect alcoholism in my patients and was prepared to argue this point in court if a compensation suit were instituted. However, the employees did not want to go to court because of their concerns about their immigration statuses and fear of losing their jobs. The company said they would use a different insecticide while insisting that they had done nothing wrong. Nothing more came of it.

The Reaganization of the government has since come to Massachusetts. There has been a systematic dismantling of activities and agencies designed to protect the health and safety of workers. In his efforts to "revitalize" the economy of the state, a Republican governor is "unburdening" industry of the very environmental protection and occupational safety reporting obligations that made it possible to find out about the poisoning of my patients.

As we will see, right-wing politics and conventional psychiatry always go hand in hand.

NINE

"*Buena suerte*, Rosa. I hope you get away with this."

I said this to myself, not actually aloud, although I believe I moved my lips as if in prayer. Not that anyone would have heard or seen. All eyes, mine included, were focused on the second-floor window of the brick tenement where a large Amerindian woman was shouting curses in Spanish. And with the fire engines and the squad cars and the ambulance and the flashing lights and crackling radios and the kids laughing—some shouting back at Rosa in mocking Spanish—no one could hear my whispered prayer.

But attention I had otherwise caught. While apparently just another curious bystander, it was me, hunched in a raincoat, *el doctor*, who had unleased this assault of Anglo authority on this woman born of the continent.

She was Uruguayan by birth, but more than half of Rosa's 40 years had been spent in the chilly grime of Chelsea. She had rid herself and her four children of the once-charming Cuban husband who when drunk would alternate among them with his beatings.

She refused welfare and cleaned houses for people who snapped orders at her, complained about an unwashed dish or a dust ball, and watched from the corners of their eyes because "you know how they are." And after scrubbing and cooking for others, she went home and scrubbed and cooked for her kids.

She had "found Jesus" at about the same time that she started to gain weight. Several nights a week and all day on Sundays, she put on a white dress and went to the Pentecostal church, the *Iglesia de Dios*, located in the decaying shell of a former synagogue. The church's name was lodged uncomfortably in the interstices of the Mogen David, whose stained glass had long since been replaced with plywood painted white.

Having been taken at age nine from her impoverished rural family to be a servant in a Montevideo household, there had been no time in her childhood for religion. She had begged to be allowed to work as a servant, and by the time she was 20, she had saved enough to come to America, to Chelsea. Healthy, beautiful, proud, optimistic, she would meet *El Norte* on its own terms and find out what life had to offer. There had been some abuse in Montevideo, which she never wanted to talk about. Now fat, poor, pious, without her abusive husband, she cooked and scrubbed and raised four children in the crowded tenement now under siege.

The oldest, Lydia, was 17 when I first got to know them. She was pretty, intense, bright, serious, and as soon as she could, she fled to a civil service secretarial job and her own apartment. But she lived in Chelsea, too, and visited several times a week and called every day. Now approaching 30, she had a more or less serious boyfriend but was in no hurry to get married. It was Lydia who would call me during a crisis.

Roberto, a couple of years younger, was inclined to get hysterical. When Rosa would become psychotic, he would lose control and, with tears of fear and screams of rage, at times come close to raising his hand to his mother, a gesture so full of the memory of his absent father that it momentarily brought looks of alarm from everyone. He was otherwise a handsome, ingratiating teenager with some tendency to exaggerate his prospects. He now has a full life in Boston and is rarely heard from.

The "kids" were separated by a decade from the older sibs. Maria and Julio were seven and six or so when I had first seen them cowering in wide-eyed terror from their raging mother. With all the talk of "shots" and hospitals and vague threats and entreaties, they might well have thought it was all about them, as if it were all their fault (as children always feel). Indeed, what coherent content there was to Rosa's screams did seem to be about them and their spoiled, selfish demands for toys at Christmas.

At 14, Maria had her first pregnancy while on cocaine. Neither she nor Rosa would consider an abortion, but the pregnancy ended in a miscarriage some weeks after a suicide attempt landed her in Lindemann. A zealous first-year resident decided that Maria was manic-depressive, since that was her mother's diagnosis, and put her on Tegretol, an anticonvulsant which the resident had learned may be effective in stabilizing a mood disorder. Tegretol, like Lithium, is more teratogenic than cocaine, more dangerous to the unborn.

I called the resident and told her to stop the drug. She refused. (Zealous first-year residents do not take orders from even senior psychiatrists who are not directly their supervisors. At the Massachusetts General Hospital, where she was in training, Tegretol was being studied as a drug for manic-depressive disorder and was very popular.) It didn't matter anyway, because Maria ran away from the hospital. A year later, she was pregnant again but fortunately had stopped using drugs, legal or otherwise.

Lisandra, Maria's daughter, is beautiful and bright, but when Rosa came home from scrubbing floors and wanted to lie down, and Maria wanted to go out to see her boyfriend, there were angry words about who did and who didn't love and care for the baby.

Julio used to be a shy, winsome, chubby little kid, cute, the kind whose cheeks one would want to squeeze between the thumb and middle finger and then imitate the little moue that resulted. Everything was scary to him, his mother's craziness, my visits, being sick with a sore throat, my looking at it with a light, and taking a culture. I often perform such unpsychiatric services in order to save a six-hour wait at an emergency ward and a $200 bill to Medicaid.

As a teenager, he has been arrested several times for breaking and entering and various thefts, probably relating to drug use. He wound up in a residential program run by the Department of Youth Services.

Rosa's craziness was perennial. Almost invariably at Christmas every few years, Lydia would call with angry tears, the anger often directed at me as if it were somehow my fault that her mother had started up again. "She threw the refrigerator off the back porch into an air shaft." Rosa was that massive and powerful, and mania has a way of doubling, maybe even tripling, one's strength.

She had tried to move the stove. "*Ni tampoco necesitamos este* [We don't need this either]," she shrieked. But in the midst of her madness, she perceived that the gas line which fueled it might be broken and could cause a problem.

There was another bit of sense to her madness, her manic fury. She was scrimping to survive, counting pennies, clothing the kids and herself from the Salvation Army recycling center, buying day-old bread and lugging canned food on sale from the supermarket a mile and a half away. Rosa was trying to keep herself and her children "alive in Christ." Her breakdown would come on His birthday because the kids, Maria and Julio, seeing the elaborate toys hyped between cartoons on TV for weeks before Christmas would, like all kids, *want* them and complain about the Salvation Army pants and shoes which Rosa more or less gift wrapped. She would feel helpless and angry and ashamed and guilty. And then she would become manic.

"You don't need those things you see on TV," she would shout in Spanish. "You don't need the TV. We don't need anything from this country. We can live on nothing. We don't need the refrigerator. I'll show you. I'll bring home the food every day. We don't need a stove. I'll show you."

After throwing the refrigerator and the TV out the window and shoving the stove a little, she would build a fire on the kitchen floor to show how they could cook their supper "like the Indians."

Screaming back that she was "*loca*," Roberto and Lydia would pour water on the fire. Lydia would call me and I would come with a pink commitment paper and a syringe filled with Prolixin decanoate, a tranquilizer which, once injected, can exert an effect for as long as a month.

I hate them both, these my most powerful of "tools." Prolixin is among the most hateful of medicines, the most disempowering, the most patronizing, the most confounding of treatment and social control. Armed with the commitment paper and the Prolixin injection, I am an agent of the state, a violator of due process. I exercise power on behalf of civility, order, and propriety. I do the dirty work of cultural repression which even the police, repressive enough in Chelsea, will not do. It's one thing to beat up a teenager in a jail cell and another to restrain him with chemicals or lock him up in four-point restraints without even the pretense of a "right to consult a lawyer." I can do that.

And I did it to Rosa. The first time I simply hospitalized her. The ambulance came, and she shook off the restraining hand of the attendant who spoke to her as many Anglos speak to Hispanics, loudly so as to be understood, condescendingly as to a child. "What's her name? Rosa? Come on, Rosa. We don't want to have to tie you down on a stretcher."

Getting the ambulance to come is easy. Getting a patient into a state psychiatric facility is a little harder. When I would call the Lindemann Center, they would want to know if I had tried to find a private bed for her, since she was covered by Medicaid. Try to find a private psychiatric bed for a Medicaid patient. First, you have to tell the admitting office the patient's story, then you have to tell the chief of the service the same story, then back to the admitting office, where they want to know what kind of insurance the patient has, and when they hear it is a Medicaid patient, they say they will find out if a bed is available and call you back. As often as not, a half hour later, they call back to say that they have no beds.

Private hospitals get more money per patient-day from Blue Cross and other private insurers than from Medicaid, so they have an unofficial, probably illegal, quota of "Medicaid beds," or they keep the Medicaid patients hanging until they are sure there will not be a private admission.

When I had the time and was not sitting with a patient threatening to run in front of the nearest truck, I would call a few private hospitals and go through this exercise. If I knew someone in the admitting office, I would simply ask, "Do you have a Medicaid bed for a female?"

But at a time like this, I would simply call Lindemann and lie. "I checked. There are no private Medicaid beds." The job of the Lindemann staff was to keep people out. They only had 40 beds and usually had over 50 patients on the ward. When they reached 60, they would simply close admissions.

Being on the ward was terrible for Rosa. There was no privacy. Designed during the era of social emancipation in the sixties, which also brought in coed college dorms, this progressive neo-asylum did not have separate sections for male and female patients. It was not uncommon for men to climb into the beds of women. The only secure environment was the "S.C.U." (pronounced "skew"), the "quiet room" where everyone was closely watched or in restraint.

For the most part, first-year psychiatric residents made up the medical staff, men and women who had been quickly socialized into using massive amounts of drugs to reduce their own anxiety, demonstrate a certain authority, and render their patients more tractable. They have little curiosity about the natural course of an acute psychosis and increasingly resort to "polypharmacy," a cocktail of different drugs. While they see *something* happening, they do not know what or why. They are not watchers but doers.

This treatment takes place within a dramatic bit of urban sculpture that looks like a piano trying to copulate with itself. A Cinderella staircase emerges gradually from engraved curvilinear lines in the sidewalk. One stumbles at first, thinking that the lines represent steps, and then stumbles again when they imperceptibly do begin to become steps. With a short rise and a two-foot tread, they cannot be climbed one at a time; one has to take a short, limping, extra little step to reach the next one. The building thereby programs disabled behavior, making one feel handicapped in the very process of entering it.

There is a certain perverse genius in the design of the building for people with poor ego boundaries. The staircase majestically rises not to but through the building onto a plaza on the opposite side. It is a plaza which actually slopes away from the building, so one feels as if on a centrifuge. One is left with the strange Kafkaesque sense that there is no way to enter this place, or to leave it.

The walls and corridors of the building are coated with the architectural signature of the famous designer who won the contract for the building, Paul Rudolph. He argued that machines could do the carving of the rocky spines for which he insists on being remembered, but the unions protested, and the whole process had to be done by hand at enormous expense to the state.

People generally like to tap a corridor wall as they walk down it as a way of assuring themselves they are not falling through a dreamlike vortex. But if you try to touch the wall of a corridor at Lindemann as you walk, your knuckles are likely to be bloodied. Since the corridors curve, one does not know where they go or when they will end, which is often in a cul-de-sac with a locked green door. These are the kinds of doors which, when panned by a movie camera, immediately evoke deeply buried instincts of horror unless we are absolutely sure that the Marx brothers are behind them.

Once I got out of the elevator to find a man shaking in terror. "What's the matter?" I asked. "I just left my doctor's office to go to the bathroom and I can't find my way back."

The whole place is hostile, disorienting, frightening. The door to the chapel is kept locked because its otherworldly, concrete forms, like the setting for a Grade B movie about the ancient Druids, attracted too many suicide attempts. Neither the cigarette smoke that layers in the stale, "conditioned" air nor that special state hospital smell of urine succeeds in humanizing the building.

This is where I would send Rosa. She would not stay very long, as she quickly accommodated to the massive doses of neuroleptics and Lithium she was given. Stiff and sedated, she would reappear at the clinic within a couple of weeks and agree to continue taking the medicine "*por ahora* [for now]," as long as I lowered the dose. Within a month or so, she would stop coming, announcing, when I called her, that she was "*muy bien* [fine]" and did not need to come any more. I tried again and again to convince her that the medicine would keep her out of the hospital, that she could take a lower dosage, that she didn't have to take the Lithium if she didn't want to have blood tests, and any other deal I could think of, including, "You don't have to take any medicine, but at least come to see me once a month." No deal. She would call me when she needed me.

A year or two later, Lydia would call again. Perhaps two or three times after the first hospitalization, I was able to convince her to accept an injection with the argument that unless she had the injection, I would send her to the hospital. It was her choice, a nonchoice dictated by the unpleasant realities of the white man's freedom. Furious, in helpless indignation, she would fling up her dress and bare her buttock to the syringe.

And each time, according to Lydia's report, she was "fine" the next day. I doubt that this was due as much to a pharmacological effect as it was to a denigration ritual, an exorcism of the proud pre-Columbian spirits that told her not to accept any more of my attention, my medicine, my arrogant, omnipotent, goddamned *kindness*. She would be "fine" for another year or two, possibly more.

But this time, it was different. Lydia said, choking with tears, that it was worse than ever. Rosa had hit her hard and physically thrown her out of the house without her coat when she had said, "Ma, you're getting *loca* again. Let me call the doctor." The neighbors had called the police, who were calling me at the same time as Lydia was. A DSS social worker had already been contacted, presumably by a neighbor, and *she* called to say that she was going to have to "place" Maria and Julio because their mother was "obviously incompetent." So it was, as if in a tragedy opening in the midst of itself, that I went to the house armed with the usual, a Prolixin injection and the "pink paper."

She would not press the buzzer that unlocked the street door. A neighbor let me in so I could knock at the door of her apartment.

"Rosa," I shouted. "*Soy yo.* It's me, Dr. Dumont." No answer, but I could hear her inside, stomping around, slamming doors. I called and knocked,

knocked and called. Finally, she shouted back, "*Vaya! No lo quiero ni su medicina* [Go away! I don't want you or your medicine]."

"Rosa, if you don't let me in, I will have to send you to the hospital."

"I'm not going to the hospital and I'm not letting you in."

I stood there for a few minutes, the neighbors watching through slightly opened doors, and then I walked away.

Did I make a decision? Might I have walked away saying to myself and everyone else, to Lydia, to the neighbors, "Well, I tried. I did my best. She doesn't want my help," thereby respecting her freedom, crazy as it was? She had not committed a crime. She was in her own home, her castle protected by centuries of Anglo-Saxon law.

I don't know if I made a decision or a decision had already been made long ago by me or others. I was swept along on the crest of a wave at the edge of a massive ocean, more massive even than the one that carried Columbus just 500 years ago. These hands, moist with the memory, scribbled my signature. The ambulance came, but the attendants refused to enter the apartment without the police. The police arrived and even with crowbars could not break open the door. Rosa had dragged a heavy dresser in front of it and was piling more furniture on top. The fire department came and, deciding against axes, placed ladders against the building so that booted, helmeted rescuers could climb through the windows.

Rosa was restrained and taken off in the snow, screaming imprecations to gods who twisted and thrashed deep within the native soil, once theirs, once hers, now blanketed by five centuries of heavy white history bearing my scrawled signature on a pink paper.

No work in this society is without its contradictions. I have always believed in "freedom" and "empowerment," and at times thought of myself as a "change agent," but much of the time my actual work has been as an agent of control.

There are nightmares in which one is trying to escape some dreadful, nameless, formless thing. One shuffles and staggers to the door, throwing oneself through, only to find oneself in the same room.

The nature of psychiatric practice, its order and direction, its purpose, its very grammar, have always reflected the social, economic, and political context in which it operates. Clinging to the trembling edge of society's identity, at the interface between normality and deviance, it may be the single most sensitive indicator of social, economic, and political forces.

As the global economy has declined, the body of theory and research, the thinking and evidence that went into social psychiatry, disappeared from the literature. Professors of psychiatry who once paid lip service to social science were replaced by a generation of pharmacologists and physiological "bench researchers" who heralded the "decade of the brain." Applied to the 1990s, this phrase was used to justify the systematic exclusion of social research from federal grants. Biological psychiatry wore a heroic "war on schizophrenia" label, which was irresistible to a population who had been socialized into believing that "breakthroughs" in the "wars" on cancer and heart disease would come from scientists doing esoteric things with exotic equipment in laboratories. The public needed only to wait and pay.

The Alliance for the Mentally Ill, representing a constituency for the most part of middle-class parents of adult "schizophrenic" children, was attracted to biological psychiatry as the alternative to the mother blaming which an earlier generation of psychoanalysts used when they (occasionally) spoke of psychosis. Biological psychiatry offered to exculpate the guilt of mothers and teased them with promise. Psychiatric residents were trained to think of psychiatric diagnoses as real disease categories referable to specific genetic defects yet to be found. "Hard science" was the serious, no-nonsense, and remunerative search for such defects.

The words *poverty* and *racism* disappeared from psychiatric journals and textbooks. It was no longer even possible to *add* the facts of psychiatric epidemiology to the putative facts of biological psychiatry. Data about the pathogenic effects of job loss and homelessness or the relationship between rates of mental illness and measures of social class were no longer relevant to a profession that had come to see illness as a function of neurotransmitters and treatment as the administration of drugs. The *correct* language of psychiatry became molecular in scale. Psychiatric trainees were no longer curious about social issues. Their training became totalitarian, with a paradigm shift that was preoccupied with the differences between things rather than their similarities.

The illusions of psychiatric thinking were the very ones that had been woven into the fabric of society's ruling ideas. Poverty itself came to be seen as the result rather than the cause of mental illness. Discussions of homelessness emphasized the numbers of mentally ill among them and implied, if not actually stated (as many did), that people became homeless *because* they were mentally ill. Reagan's construction of this was more straightforward: the homeless were there because they *wanted* to be there.

Social problems became blanched of social reality. The universe was cut and dried to fit the categories of a narrow-minded scientific frame of reference that was happy to become the handmaiden of the Right.

In the spring of 1992, the administrator of the Alcohol, Drug Abuse and Mental Health Administration blurted out his contention that the violence in the "jungles" of our cities could be explained on the basis of male primate hyperaggressive and hypersexual instincts. When the racism of this was pointed out, he apologized and accepted a "demotion" to the directorship of the National Institute of Mental Health. This was the same physician who had reported an interest in finding biological markers in children as young as five years of age who might in the future become violent.

In 1992, the sparks of social psychiatry and community mental health were finally stamped out in Massachusetts in the guise of privatization, the sacrament for the last living god, the Market.

Health care came to be parasitized by a system of investment capital crumbling under the sheer weight of profits built on credit manipulations. The ancient, time-honored means by which capital rejuvenated itself through a war did not work anymore. The crumbs of profitability in basic human needs had to be swept up when there was nothing else left to invest in. Privatization was the means to repudiate the ill and needy as a public and shared responsibility. It was justified on the basis of faith in the rationality and vigor of the "laws" of the market, the guidance of an "invisible hand." A leaner and more efficient private sector was to replace the public one.

But there were profiteers. "Nonprofit" hospitals in Boston continued to build billion-dollar towers long after health planners argued that such construction was unnecessary and inflationary. Despite the limited clinical utility of MRI machines and comparable equipment, they were purchased with reckless abandon and used routinely. There was neither the need nor the money for these buildings and equipment. In fact, while funds were being spent on construction and the purchase of expensive technology, growing numbers of nurses, aides, laundry workers, janitors, and secretaries were being laid off in "cost-cutting" measures. The decision to lay off personnel and to build billion-dollar towers is made by trustees who collectively represent the banking, insurance, and real estate interests of Boston. The billions for these investments must be borrowed at prevailing interest rates from . . . the banking, insurance, and real estate interests of Boston.

What appears to be merely inflationary health care is actually a systematic means for the sustenance of credit-based profiteering. Nonprofit institutions are the conduit of money from a shrinking and overwhelmed middle class to banks, which are far from nonprofit.

Privatization eventually came to mental health. One of the features of this period of economic decadence is a mythology about "management" which suggests that a certain kind of "rational" decision making will increase productivity even when nothing is being produced.

In the nonprofit setting, managers wear the same mantle of hegemony and self-importance as they do in the investor-owned setting. They insist on high salaries, private offices, secretaries, and, of course, computers. When cost cutting becomes necessary, they do not lower their own salaries or bonuses and they often actually increase their expenditures on computers as part of a "rationalized" process of budget cutting. They will arrange for clinicians to be laid off and productivity demands exacted from the remaining ones. This is not unlike a ship without fuel whose captain begins to pull up the planks of its own deck to throw into the furnace.

"Productivity" is an interesting word in a health care setting. It implies that medical and mental health treatment can be provided and measured like cars and television sets, so that more "units" are produced at less cost. There is no such thing as a unit of mental health, and even if it were possible to measure, managers would not be interested. What they care about is the number of billable direct-service units of time. The definition of mental health becomes a matter of how much money can be generated from public or private funds.

There are consequences of this for the community, for the patients, and for the clinical providers themselves. Since such activities as identifying the extent and sources of lead poisoning, talking to occupational health specialists, or attending community meetings are not billable, there is a systematic disincentive to become involved in these or other activities of primary prevention.

Since home visits or prolonged individual psychotherapy are not as remunerative as short-term, drug-assisted encounters, there is a tendency to make contacts as time limited and medically oriented as possible. This includes such irrational constraints as limiting treatment to seven sessions for a child who has been brutalized. The economic infrastructure of clinic practice actually programs unethical behavior. Psychotherapeutic as well as community health issues become irrelevant. Expensive, intrusive, medically-dominated interventions are encouraged.

In addition, since missed sessions for canceled appointments or "no-shows" are not reimbursable, managers encourage or demand that intake decisions focus on the selection of clients who are predictable and reliable about keeping appointments. Those whose lives are disorganized by mental illness, cultural disruptions, or the vicissitudes of poverty, i.e., *those most in need of care*, will not be accepted for treatment.

It does not matter whether a clinician decides to base his or her decisions on clinical need. If managers provide a weekly score of productivity based on billable hours, and if that score is somehow related to pay scales or job security, the clinician will *unconsciously* modify his or her behavior to increase that score. It is a classic operant conditioning technique not lost on business schools.

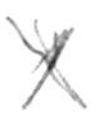

Privatization, productivity requirements, managed care, or incentive practice amount to the deprofessionalization of health care. Clinicians become the mere agents of an economic system or bits in a computer system. Marx and Engels described the "alienation" of human labor that comes with capitalism. Workers become increasingly alienated from their own labor and eventually from themselves. The privatization of health care involves the alienation and proletarianization of health workers and inevitably contributes to the destruction of their own health.

There is evidence that when an activity is rewarded on the basis of piecework rather than salaried, workers experience higher rates of stress-related illnesses such as peptic ulcers, coronary heart disease, and hypertension. Mutual cooperation and support is also systematically destroyed in such environments, so that the very protections against stress are dismantled by the same processes that induce stress. Managers in privatized clinics discourage "excess" time spent in case conferences or in-service training. Coffee breaks and lunch periods are rigidly defined, so informal peer-oriented discussions are replaced by strictly limited, bureaucratically defined, and hierarchically dominated conferences that satisfy "utilization review" guidelines. Instead of talking about the real problems experienced with a client and the personal, family, and social dynamics underlying them, mindless, meaningless dialogues about the "correct" DSM-III-R diagnosis take place. Instead of clinicians getting some understanding from co-workers about their real worries in a particular case, there is a clipped and routinized decision tree about the precise number of treatment sessions projected.

A managerial imperative exists in such environments that not only confirms its own necessity and importance but carries an implicit contempt for purely clinical points of view. The more a clinical perspective is insisted upon, the less relevant it is thought to be.

In the sixties, at the height of the community mental health movement, it would have been inconceivable for financial considerations to be thought more compelling than clinical ones. Somehow an MBA is now considered "higher" than an MSW, and mental health professionals have been disempowered. They rarely feel the right and never the obligation to challenge the authority and perquisites of business managers.

In one notable exception to this, in 1991, the physicians employed by an HMO, the Harvard Community Health Plan, went on strike to protest the "assembly-line medicine" demanded by a manager. The strike was successful, and the manager was forced to leave. Such events are rare in a mental health setting and, with privatization and the associated destruction of public service unions, are even less likely.

The administrators of public mental health agencies are now chosen to justify cost cutting with the jargon of the marketplace. In Massachusetts, the commissioner of mental health spoke of "right-sizing" instead of downsizing and closing of mental hospitals. The laying off of state personnel from outpatient clinics such as the one in Chelsea was justified on the basis of our serving the "worried well." This was a term used to describe people who had not previously experienced prolonged or repeated psychiatric hospitalizations. In Chelsea, it included such people as refugees from Central America who were victims of torture, children who had been sexually abused, women who had been raped, and, from time to time, the rapists themselves. We saw families devastated by alcoholism, unemployment, or homelessness, and old men and women whose dementia and isolation exposed themselves and their neighbors to the risk of fire through a forgotten cigarette or gas jet. These were the "worried well."

The work I did in Chelsea was demanding, but it was not "hard." I rarely felt exhausted or overwhelmed, primarily because I worked in a setting of mutual respect and support. I frequently tell students and trainees who will one day be looking for work as mental health professionals that the single most important issue in a prospective work place is the way people treat one another. If there is a sense that communication is circular rather than linear and hierarchical, that people talk to one another, there is the possibility of job satisfaction. If on the other hand, disciplines are tightly drawn and hierarchies dominate, so that one speaks in an atmosphere of refined fearfulness, it does not matter how high the pay or status; the work will be draining and demoralized.

One of the hidden features of American culture is the fantasy of nonbelonging. At some level, every one of us in any social situation, at work, play, or prayer, expects a tap on the shoulder and the question "What the hell are *you* doing here?" Ultimately, we feel that we do not belong in adult society itself, as if the mask of maturity, civility, and self-control will be ripped from our face to reveal the trembling child within. A mental health setting deserving of the name has to be set against the cultural mythology of provisional membership in humanity. However feebly, it must function as a reminder that more than 90 percent of human existence on earth has been in the context of hunter-gatherer tribes in which the welfare of one was the same as the welfare of all, in which membership and belonging were inevitable and unavoidable.

To be mentally ill is to feel one's membership in society up for question. It is to be marginal, deviant, outside. It has always been functional for fragmented and fluid social systems to identify and persecute deviants, who serve as the territorial markers for a false and fleeting sense of identity. We are not *them*—Jews, witches, communists, psychotics—we are the *not them.*

A mental health clinic cannot be expected to function as a model of utopia, but it can at least try to minimize the forces of alienation and mute somewhat the discords of a society that is endlessly exclusive and harshly rejecting. These are not technical issues of psychotherapy or medical management; they are human ones. It does not matter how expertly trained, how sensitive or competent the professionals are. If they work in a rigid, authoritarian, or insecure environment, they cannot perform a mental health function. Clients in a mental health clinic immediately perceive the way people treat each other and will always identify with the most vulnerable, the least secure, the first to be excluded.

This is why the managerial demands of productivity are so inappropriate to mental health. They frustrate the essence of social psychiatry and community mental health, by which I mean mental health not just *in* the community but *of* the community itself. Accountability in such a setting is not to a business manager or to a computer program, but to one another and, ultimately, to the community, perhaps even to the *idea* of community.

Even through the distorting lenses of hindsight, I cannot say that such an environment existed at the Chelsea clinic. But we were, at least, struggling with it and, at times, seemed to approach it.

The struggle came to an end abruptly when the governor laid off 800 state-salaried mental health professionals working in outpatient settings. The clinics were to be downsized and privatized. For all intents and purposes, the Chelsea Community Counseling Center ceased to exist.

I chose to remain in the public sector and have been working in a state hospital. For me, this represents the closing of a circle, a return to the place where social psychiatry began.

I had devoted a career to a vision of mental health practice quite different from that of the state hospital. But it was a vision that could only be realized in the wider field of a society struggling against its own inequities. And now, as if there were no end to the capacity to regress, Massachusetts and other states are in the process of closing their state hospitals. We are returning to a pre-Dorothea Dix situation in which the mentally ill can once again be found in shelters and jails and on the streets.

This is part of the systematic destruction of a social infrastructure for the urban poor. The welfare system is being dismantled at the moment when more and more helpless human beings are being generated by a heartless and brutal social system. Child welfare agencies, with all their contradictions, are being devastated as more and more abused and neglected children are forced upon them. We are laying off teachers and closing schools while we open more prisons. This is the legacy left to its children of a society in decline: the disruption of the gossamer network of mutual responsibility that we call "community." It is what happened to the *Ik*.

It was not easy to say goodbye to Chelsea. After 16 years, I had become connected in ways I would not have guessed. You do not know how deep your roots are until they are pulled out. I would walk down the street and be waved at by people in windows. The children of patients I had known as children would pull on my coat and giggle.

When I began to say goodbye, it felt like a slow tearing. I had to say goodbye to Rosa and Queenie and Lorraine and Arnold and Alfredo and Vicky and Ramón and Robert (now dead) and hundreds of others. I had to say goodbye to a staff that felt, after years of being together, like a family: a functional one, a group of people who had learned to work together, to rely on one another, to like one another, to *trust* one another. We had looked forward to seeing each other.

I had to say goodbye to streets whose crooks and crevices I had begun to know. I think I could walk them blindfolded, finding my way by their texture.

I had to say goodbye to my professional *raison d'être*, community psychiatry. From now on, it would be just a succession of jobs—not nothing these days and not bad ones either, but just jobs.

On one of the last afternoons I spent in Chelsea, with spring softening the edges of the city and dormant smells beginning to stir, I got a whiff of something familiar. It was the scent of white port from Joe's breath as he was shuffling down the street. The drink was not, as he had once carefully explained, to be confused with port wine, a more delicate and natural distillate of grapes that had once clustered along the Minho of Portugal. This was a rock-gut liquor, sweet, potent, artificial—the stuff of bottle gangs, the lowest level anodyne of the streets, below even Thunderbird and Muscatel.

I called after him, "Joe, I have to tell you something. I may not see you again. I was laid off."

"Laid off? How can they lay you off? You're a doctor."

"I'm a state employee. The governor laid me off. The clinic is going to close."

"Where do I get my pills?" He meant Dilantin for his seizures. He routinely asked for Valium and I routinely denied his request. It was a ritual.

"You'll have to go to the clinic at Lindemann."

"I won't go to that dump." After a pause, "What are you going to do?"

"I'm getting a job at Metropolitan State Hospital. But that's going to close in a few months. They are privatizing everything."

He laughed.

"What's funny?" I asked.

"A state is really going downhill when they start laying off garbage men."

"What do you mean?"

"You've been taking care of garbage. Me. Waste. They throw things away. People, too. You're supposed to keep the garbage off the streets."

"Recycle?"

"That's what you want to think. No, just keeping the garbage off the streets. That's what they paid you for. And they can't even afford that now. So the garbage piles up."

"I never thought of you as garbage, Joe."

"I'm garbage, something they don't need and don't want. And guess what? You're garbage, too, now."

I did not feel offended.

REFERENCES

INTRODUCTION

Brenner, H. *Mental Illness and the Economy.* Cambridge, Mass.: Harvard University Press, 1973.

Brown, G. et al. "Life Events and Psychiatric Disorder." *Psychological Medicine,* 3(2), 1973.

Dumont, M. "A Diagnostic Parable. A Review of DSM-III-R." *Readings* (American Orthopsychiatric Association), 2(4), 1987.

Dumont, M. "Is Mental Health Possible Under Our Economic System?" *Psychiatric Opinion,* 14(3), 1977.

Fried, M. "Grieving for a Lost Home." In L. Duhl, ed., *The Urban Condition.* New York: Basic Books, 1963.

Kagan, J. "On Class Differences and Early Development." In V. Denenberg, ed., *Education of the Infant and Young Child.* New York: Academic Press, 1970.

Seligman, M. *Helplessness.* San Francisco: Freeman, 1975.

Turnbull, C. *The Mountain People.* New York: Simon and Schuster, 1972.

CHAPTER 1

Deutsch, A. *The Shame of the States.* New Hampshire: Ayer, 1948.

Dumont, M. *The Absurd Healer: Perspectives of a Community Psychiatrist.* New York: Viking (Compass), 1970.

Dumont, M. "The Junkie As Political Enemy." *American Journal of Orthopsychiatry,* 3(4), 1973.

Jacoby, R. *The Repression of Psychoanalysis.* New York: Basic Books, 1983.

CHAPTER 2

Caplan, G. *Principles of Preventive Psychiatry.* New York: Basic Books, 1964.

Caudill, W. et al. *Architecture for the Community Mental Health Center.* New York: Mental Health Materials Center, 1967.

Dumont, M. "Tavern Culture: The Sustenance of Homeless Men." *American Journal of Orthopsychiatry,* 38(5), 1967.

Dumont, M., and Aldrich, C. "Family Care After a Thousand Years: A Crisis in the Tradition of St. Dymphna." *American Journal of Psychiatry,* 119(2), 1962.

Hollingshead, A., and Redlich, F. *Social Class and Mental Illness.* New York: John Wiley, 1958.

Jacobs, J. *The Death and Life of the Great American City.* New York: Random House, 1961.

Jones, M. *Maturation of the Therapeutic Community.* New York: Human Sciences Press, 1976.

Leighton, A. et al. *The Sterling County Study of Psychiatric Disorder and Sociocultural Environment.* New York: Basic Books, 1959.

Lindemann, E. "The Symptomatology and Management of Acute Grief." *American Journal of Psychiatry,* 101(141), 1944.

Pasamanick. B. et al. "Socioeconomic Status and Some Precursors of Neuropsychiatric Disorder." *American Journal of Orthopsychiatry,* 26(594), 1936.

Smith, M. et al. *Benefits of Psychotherapy.* Baltimore: Johns Hopkins University Press, 1980.

Srole, L. et al. *Mental Health in the Metropolis.* New York: Harper, 1962.

CHAPTER 3

Dumont, M. "The Changing Face of Professionalism." *Social Policy*, 1(1), 1970.

Dumont, M. "Civil Commitment of the Addict." In L.R.S. Simmons and M. B. Gold, eds., *Discrimination and the Addict.* Beverly Hills: International Yearbook of Drug Addiction, 1973.

Dumont, M. "CODAP: The Monster Masquerading As A Windmill." *Rough Times*, March 1974.

Dumont, M. "Down the Bureaucracy." *Trans-Action*, 7(12), 1970.

Dumont, M. "Drug Problems and Their Treatment." In *The American Handbook of Psychiatry, Vol. 2.* Rev. Ed. New York: Basic Books, 1974.

Dumont, M. "Government As Dada." *Trans-Action*, 8(7), 1971.

Dumont, M. "Mainlining America: Why the Young Use Drugs." *Social Policy* 2, no. 4 (1971).

Dumont, M. "The Politics of Drugs." *Social Policy*, 2(4), 1972.

Dumont, M. "Self-Help Treatment Programs." *American Journal of Psychiatry*, 131(6), 1974.

Dumont, M. "Technology and the Treatment of Addiction." In S. Fisher and A. Freedman, eds., *Opiate Addiction: Origins and Treatment.* Washington, D.C.: Winston, 1973.

Parenti, M. *Make-Believe Media.* New York: St. Martins, 1992.

CHAPTER 4

Needleman, H. "Deficits in Psychological and Classroom Performance of Children with Elevated Lead Levels." *New England Journal of Medicine*, 300(689), 1979.

CHAPTER 5

Brown, G. et al. "Life Events and Psychiatric Disorder," 1973.

Calhoun, J. "Population Density and Social Pathology." *Scientific American*, 206(139), 1962.

Kagan, J. "On Class Differences and Early Development," 1970 op. cit.

Seligman, M. *Helplessness*, 1975 op. cit.

CHAPTER 6

Alberman, E. "Disabilities in Survivors of Low Birth Weight." *Archives of Diseases in Children*, 60(913), 1985.

Babel, I. "The Palace of Motherhood." In *You Must Know Everything*. New York: Farrar, Strauss, Geroux, 1966.

Behrman, R. "Preventing Low Birthweight: A Pediatric Perspective." *Journal of Pediatrics*, 107(6), 1985.

Birch, H., and Gussow, J. *Disadvantaged Children: Health, Nutrition and School Failure*. New York: Harcourt, Brace and World, 1970.

Bolton, F. "Child Maltreatment Risk Among Adolescent Mothers." *American Journal of Orthopsychiatry*, 50(3), 1980.

Centers for Disease Control. "Effects of Restrictions on Medicaid Funding for Abortions." *Morbidity and Mortality Weekly Report*, 29(22), 1980.

Kinnard, E., and Klerman, L. "Teenage Parenting and Child Abuse." *American Journal of Orthopsychiatry*, 50(3), 1980.

Phipps Yonas, S. "Teenage Pregnancy and Motherhood." *American Journal of Orthopsychiatry*, 30(3), 1980.

Preventing Low Birthweight. Study of the Committee of the National Institute of Medicine. Washington, D.C.: National Academy Press, 1985.

CHAPTER 8

Drummond, H. "Empires Born, Bred and Dead of Lead." In *Dr. Drummond's Spirited Guide to Health Care in a Dying Empire.* New York: Grove (Black Cat), 1980.

Dumont, M. "Community Organization and the Prevention of Lead Poisoning." *Health-Pac Bulletin,* 13(2), 1982.

Dumont, M. "The Non-Specificity of Mental Illness." *American Journal of Orthopsychiatry,* 54(2), 1984.

Needleman, H. "Deficits in Psychological and Classroom Performance of Children with Elevated Lead Levels," 1979.

CHAPTER 9

Dumont, M. "In Bed Together in the Market: Psychiatry and the Pharmaceutical Industry."*American Journal of Orthopsychiatry,* 60(4), 1990.

Dumont, M. "Psychotoxicology: The Return of the Mad Hatter." *Social Science and Medicine,* 29(2), 1989.

Hamilton, H., and Hardy, H. *Industrial Toxicology.* 3rd ed. Acton, Mass.: Publishing Sciences Group, 1974.

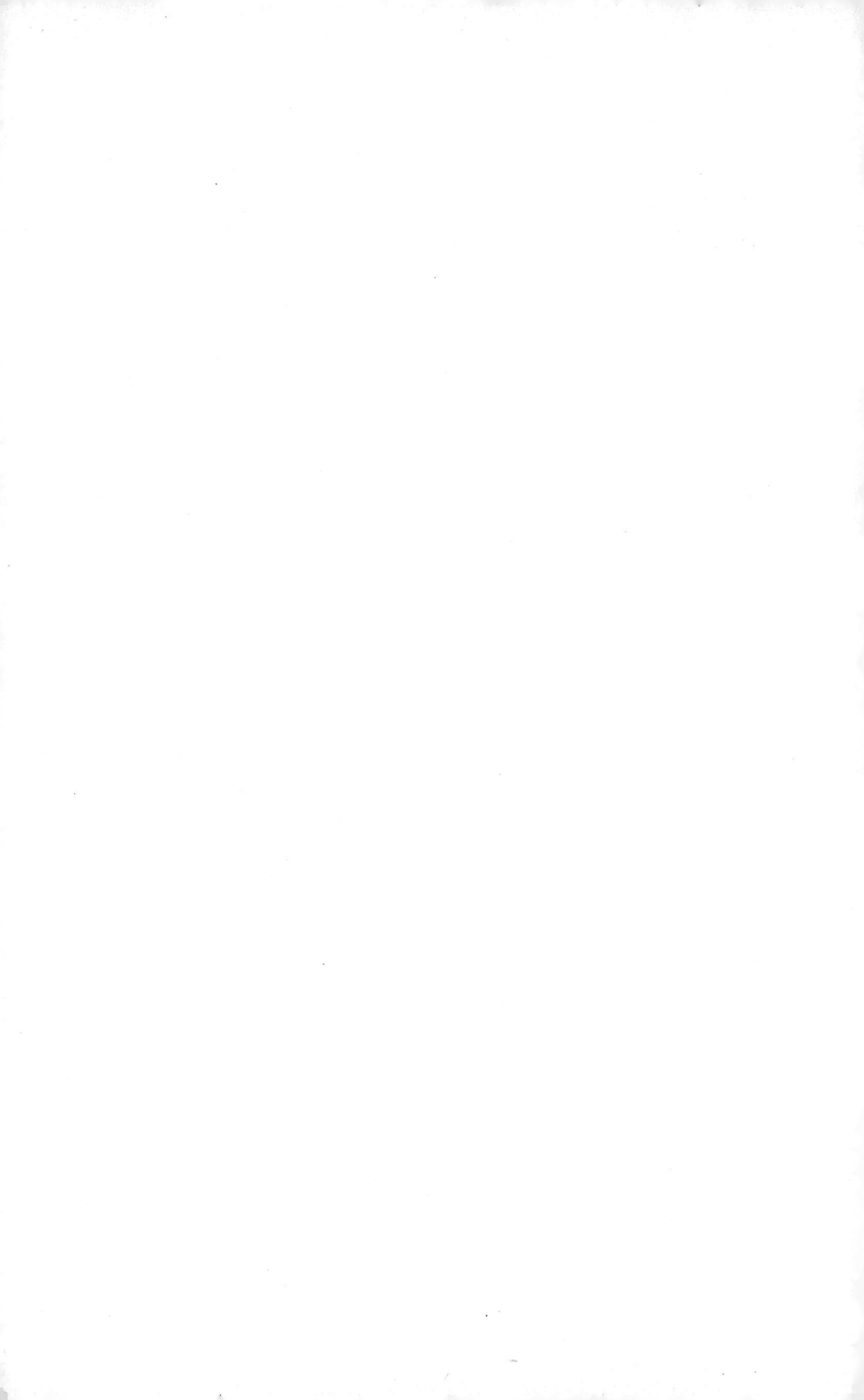